The A to Z Refe[...]
Syndromes and Inherited Disorders

The A-Z Reference Book of Syndromes and Inherited Disorders

A manual for health, social and education workers

Patricia Gilbert

Visiting Senior Lecturer
Warwick University
UK

CHAPMAN & HALL
London · Glasgow · New York · Tokyo · Melbourne · Madras

Published by Chapman & Hall, 2–6 Boundary Row, London SE1 8HN

Chapman & Hall, 2–6 Boundary Row, London SE1 8HN, UK

Blackie Academic & Professional, Wester Cleddens Road, Bishopbriggs, Glasgow G64 2NZ, UK

Chapman & Hall, 29 West 35th Street, New York NY10001, USA

Chapman & Hall Japan, Thomson Publishing Japan, Hirakawacho Nemoto Building, 6F, 1-7-11 Hirakawa-cho, Chiyoda-ku, Tokyo 102, Japan

Chapman & Hall Australia, Thomas Nelson Australia, 102 Dodds Street, South Melbourne, Victoria 3205, Australia

Chapman & Hall India, R. Seshadri, 32 Second Main Road, CIT East, Madras 600 035, India

First edition 1993

Co-published in the United States with Singular Publishing Group Inc., San Diego, California

© 1993 Chapman & Hall

Typeset in 10/12 Palatino by Expo Holdings Sdn. Bhd.

Printed in Great Britain by St Edmundsbury Press, Bury St. Edmunds

ISBN 0 412 47130 2   1 56593 046 0 (USA only)

A catalogue record for this book is available from the British Library

Library of Congress Cataloging-in-Publication data to follow

Contents

Foreword

More often than not, my heart sinks when I know I am to see a family with a child who has a 'syndrome'. It sinks because it is highly likely that I will not understand the cause of the syndrome, that there will be no specific treatment, that the outlook (particularly in newly described syndromes) may be unknown, and, most importantly, the parents will ask me sensible and pertinent questions that I cannot answer. Only if I have special expertise in the disorder, or group of disorders, will I be able to help the child as I would wish. Clearly I cannot have expertise in, or knowledge of, even a fraction of the over 2000 syndromes now described.

My difficulties are, I am sure, shared to a greater or lesser extent by all who may be involved in counselling, or caring for, those handicapped by a 'syndrome'. Many who will be responsible for providing for the child's needs, and to whom the parents may turn, may not even have any background medical knowledge. This book, written simply and concisely and in non-technical language gives just the sort of information needed. It will be a boon to those working in Child Health in the community, in Social Services and in schools.

To cover more than a small selection of the known 'syndromes' is clearly impracticable, and to be always up-to-date with the latest 'discovery' in such a rapidly moving field is impossible. Dr. Gilbert, with her extensive experience, has chosen wisely, and much of the practical information that she gives will not date. Patients, parents and professionals will have reason to be grateful to her for having compiled this compendium on a difficult and important topic.

Professor Dame June Lloyd

Preface

Syndromes are part of everyday diagnosis today. The number described seems to increase weekly. Hitherto, few were known or documented accurately. Just what are these conditions so labelled?

The *Oxford English Dictionary* defines a 'syndrome' as 'a concurrence of several symptoms in a disease; a set of such concurrent symptoms'. Put in simpler terms, a 'syndrome' can be described as a specific collection of signs and symptoms which, when put together, form a recognizable pattern which can be seen to be repeated in another individual.

There are now over 2000 of these syndromes recorded. Some are incredibly rare, others uncommon, whilst others in comparison are relatively frequently seen. For example, in the latter group is Down's syndrome – well-known to most people – with a general incidence of one in approximately every 800 births. Examples of the rarer syndromes are Hunter's and Hurler's syndromes. Both of these syndromes are only found in one child in 100 000. Few doctors, nurses, teachers or social workers (unless their work happened to be with handicapped children or adults) will have seen more than a handful of such syndromes. Nevertheless, with the ever-increasing number of syndromes being classified, many of these professionals could well be seeing several people with a specific syndrome during their working life.

At some time during the lives of people who have a definable syndrome, and most commonly in childhood, help in some form, be it medical, nursing, social or educational, will be needed. In the early days, parents will need support, advice and counselling in order to come to terms with their child's disability, as well as more practical aspects of care. Later in the child's life, social workers and educationalists become involved. All these professionals need accurate knowledge of each specific syndrome if they are to be fully effective in their support of families.

In this book, a small number of the known syndromes, alphabetically listed, are described. Each section gives guidelines on the practical aspects of help that can be given. Any one of the disciplines of medicine, nursing, social work or education may be involved, but in many cases all four disciplines will have a part to play. Many of the syndromes have self-help groups which have been set up over the years, most frequently by parents who themselves have a child with the specific disorder. Contact points for these self-help groups are to be found at the end of each appropriate section. A basic outline of genetics is given in **appendix A**. The effects of a handicapping condition on the individual, the family and society in general are also discussed separately. Comprehensive cross-indexing is included to help the reader towards the correct syndrome. For instance, all syndromes having short stature as a characteristic are listed together, as are those syndromes in which a squint might be a factor.

It is hoped that this book will prove to be of value to all professionals who are concerned with the care of handicapped children. It has been difficult to limit the number of syndromes described to a manageable minimum. The main criteria that have been involved in this choice are two-fold. Firstly, that the syndrome will result in long-term, and in many cases lifelong, problems of one kind or another, either mental or physical. Secondly, that help is available which can alleviate some of the problems and improve the quality of life. The author will be pleased to receive comments and suggestions as to possible further inclusions at a later date.

Finally, my thanks are due to all the many children with a 'syndrome', and their parents, with whom I have had the privilege to work over the years.

Acknowledgements

My thanks are due to a number of people who have given encouragement and help with the writing of this book. In particular, Dr. Terry Billington has given unstintingly of her time and expertise in reading the manuscript. Without her medical and physiotherapy skills much would have been lost. Dr. Peter Farndon also has found time in his exceedingly busy life to give advice on the genetics appendix, and for this I am in his debt. But it must be emphasized that any errors in the text are entirely my own.

Much gratitude is also felt to Professor June Lloyd for writing the foreword, and I would like to thank her again for her kind words and sentiments.

Finally, my thanks to my husband who has guided me successfully through the minefields of word-processing with patience and cheerfulness.

The effects of handicap

Our genetic inheritance colours all our life. The medical conditions passed down the family line will affect our daily lives as surely as does our height, the colour of our skin and our potential for low or high ability. And when a syndrome, or specifically inherited condition, is part of our family tree, these effects can be very great indeed. Our family, our friends and the wider society in which we live will also be affected by our genetic inheritance to a greater or lesser degree. These effects will not cease when childhood is outgrown. The whole of our adult life will be altered, for better or worse.

Between 15% and 20% of adults suffer from some chronic condition which has a bearing on some, or all, of their daily living. Some of these problems are due, of course, to reasons other than inherited disease. Infection and environmental factors all play their part. But it is thought that some 16% of all babies born alive have some defect, many small and insignificant, at birth. About half of these will have a condition that will give rise to functional problems of one kind or another, throughout their lives. So this aspect of life will have an impact on very many people, whether directly in a day-to-day manner, in the work environment or merely by chance encounter.

Obviously the greatest effect of an inherited disease will be felt by each individual having the specific condition. Every baby has the same basic needs of warmth, food, love and a sense of belonging. The first two of these necessities will be met in all but the most unfortunate of babies. (Although problems of adequate nutrition may cause difficulties in some babies, however, as a result of their genetic inheritance, quite apart from economic factors.) It is love and, later, a sense of belonging that some severely disabled babies can lack. Mothers, who have waited for nine long months for the arrival of a perfect baby, can be distraught at the sight of a handicapped newcomer. Careful and sensitive handling of the situation, by those caring for the mother and baby, will be needed. The majority of mothers, under these circumstances, will accept their baby with love, but a few may take time to come to terms with the unexpected problems facing them. Fortunately relatively few mothers completely reject their handicapped child.

Later in the child's life, problems of acceptance can also occur. This is especially true of the child who has an inherited disorder needing much daily – and possibly nightly – care. Parents can become completely exhausted by the unremitting and inevitable demands of their handicapped child. Child abuse, in any one of a number of guises, may occur, and must be remembered as a possibility under these circumstances. Doctors, nurses and social workers, and also teachers when schooldays are reached, should all be aware of the strain under which the parents of a handicapped child are living. Help, be it practical, financial or by means of respite care should be made available before the burdens become intolerable.

A further basic need of childhood, and indeed throughout life, is the need to be able to continue to learn. Children with handicaps can often miss out on this vital aspect of normal living. To avoid this, the precise diagnosis of his/her condition must be made initially. Following on from this, assessment of the effects on various functions, vision, hearing, mobility to mention just a few, will be needed. Only then can a specific programme of learning, at whatever basic level, be organized. It is important that the exact nature of the disability is diagnosed early. Vital stages of learning can be missed by this oversight. For example, a baby born with a profound hearing loss will rarely, if ever, be able to speak unless the hearing problem is recognized, and appropriate treatment and training given. Similarly, there are 22 children in every 100 000 in the UK who are registered as blind. These children may have a little residual vision, but this will be too little for the learning process to proceed normally. So suitable educational facilities for learning by methods involving touch must be organized. These are but two examples of the ways in which inherited disease, or a syndrome, can affect an individual's capacity for one of the basic needs of life.

Parents, too, should be carefully advised on what activities are most suitable for the developmental age of their child. Chronological age, in many syndromes which have a degree of mental retardation as part of the symptomatology, is no guide to the stage of development the child has reached. For example, a child with Down's syndrome is frequently behind his/her contemporaries in many aspects of mobility. His/her walking will be delayed due to the almost universal hypotonia found in Down's children. So it is inadvisable for parents to buy toys which are designed for children with early onset of this particular skill. Later, as the child with this handicap falls further behind his/her peers, toys and activities will need to be geared to his/her mental abilities rather than to his/her physical age.

A further aspect of life with an inherited handicapping condition is the possible need for frequent hospital admissions. This can have two major effects on the life of the individual child. He/she will be away for, sometimes long, periods of time from his/her immediate family and friends. This can loosen the ties of everyday involvement with work and play. For the older child, when school days are a reality, lessons are also missed unless there can be a close liaison with school, home and hospital. During an acute bout of illness, school work obviously cannot be considered. But during convalescence, time can usefully, and happily, be spent catching up with class work. This especially applies to children with such conditions as cystic fibrosis and osteogenesis imperfecta, for example. In these two conditions (and there are many others) hospitalization can be a recurrent necessity. All efforts to maintain contact with family and friends should be made.

Finally, when considering the effects of handicap on a particular child, appreciation of him/her as an individual must never be forgotten. It is all too easy to talk down to a child in a wheelchair who has perhaps an added speech or hearing problem. It is important, and especially as the teenage years are reached, that these young people should be involved in decisions as to their future if at all possible. Whether later schooling should be in a special school, or in a mainstream school with added resources involves the child as much as – or perhaps more than – the parents. Choices must be worked out with the child's comments and feelings an important part of the discussion.

Careers, if applicable, must also be a joint decision between child, parent and advisor. Some handicaps will of course prevent any of the more active careers being pursued. But many conditions can allow the sufferer to work alongside their peers with no such disability. Extra consideration for particular activities, such as ramps for those people with a mobility problem, extra light for poor vision, for instance, may be needed. These, and many other possible complications, must be thought through carefully. But the wishes of the young person should be an important part of the final decision.

To summarize how parents and professionals involved in the care of a child with a handicap can make life as normal as possible:

1. All efforts should be made to learn as much as possible about the condition from which the child is suffering. Knowing what difficulties the child has to overcome will be half-way to helping him/her to cope with his/her disability. For instance, try to see what life is really like with only central, or 'tunnel', vision by blinkering off the range of side vision with an anorak hood. Crossing the road safely becomes twice as difficult, and people coming up quietly behind you can be fairly frightening. Again, tie one arm behind you to find out just how difficult it is to perform many everyday activities with only one functioning arm. These, of course, are gross examples, and ones easily replicated. How much more difficult is it to understand the problems encountered by children with poor cognitive abilities whose surroundings make little sense to them. But this is just what carers should be trying to do, so that the best possible help can be given.
2. Find out how the specific condition may progress. What will the child be doing and feeling when, say, five years have passed. Syndromes and other inherited disorders vary greatly in the way they progress – some may reach a plateau and stay there for many years, whilst

others regrettably progress rapidly. Many syndromes have self-help groups, often started by parents who themselves have a child with the particular condition. Here other sufferers from the same, or similar, condition can correspond or even meet to compare notes on various problems and how best to overcome them. Much information can be gained on practical aspects of daily living, benefits obtainable as well as friendship, from such sources.

3. All parents have ambitions for their children. When their son or daughter has been found to have a specific handicapping condition these ambitions will have to be substantially altered. Sometimes, with a severely affected child, the outlook for life itself is limited. With yet other serious disorders, parents will be forced to accept that only the most minimal of self-help skills will ever be attained. This can be devastatingly difficult for even the most mature and sympathetic parent, but from the child's point of view it is of immense significance that the adjustment is made. Realistic boundaries can then be set. Here again, sympathetic help from others in similar circumstances can be of enormous value.

4. Children who need hospitalization can be prepared for these events. Finding out about admission procedures, what clothing to take, toys allowed and many other day-to-day events can do much to alleviate the fear of the unknown. A positive attitude in the parents themselves to the outcome of the perhaps extended and painful procedures will serve to minimize the upsets of admissions to hospital. Whilst the child is actually in hospital, regular visits with small gifts, photographs of family and day-to-day updates of home news can do much to negate feelings of isolation.

Close liaison with medical and nursing staff regarding the type and length of proposed treatments can help parents explain to their child what is likely to happen to them within the next day or two. Parents are welcome in most hospitals nowadays to be with their child when at all possible during treatment. Mothers, for example, are able to be with their child immediately before an anaesthetic, and also to be at their child's side when he/she 'comes round'.

5. Diets necessary to the well-being of the handicapped child can be at times unpalatable and different from the food their friends are eating. These can be made as palatable as possible and explanations given to friends about the necessity for any restrictions.

6. Finally it must be remembered that children who have a syndrome are twice as likely to have some behavioural disorder as their peers. This is in addition to the effects of the disorder itself. If parents are warned of this, and counselled as to how best to avoid these problems, the incidence of outbursts will be reduced to a minimum.

These then are some of the aspects an inherited disorder can have on the individual child. But what about the parents, who, instead of their hoped-for perfect son or daughter, are faced with a baby who, in addition to looking 'different', has the prospect of needing special, continuing care for many years?

The immediate reaction to the birth of an obviously handicapped baby is one of shock and disbelief. Both partners will need sensitive, and ongoing, sympathy and counselling if they are both to accept their baby as he/she is. They must be allowed to grieve, for the birth of handicapped child is surely a bereavement, as is a still-birth. All the hopes and aspirations for a perfect, healthy baby are dashed in one brief moment. Parents need time and space to come to terms with their loss. All the usual grief reactions will be there – disbelief, anger, guilt, depression and finally acceptance. These stages will, of course, vary from person to person. Some mothers will find it easy to love and care for their baby, whilst others will find this a traumatic ordeal that has to be worked at for some time. The father, too, must not be forgotten. He may be very supportive, but he, as well, will need to work through his disappointment. Thankfully the vast majority of parents come to terms with the outcome of the pregnancy and continue, often for many years, to love and care for their handicapped child. Later, as the child grows and possibly becomes more and more demanding of the mother's time and energies, the marriage may be put under severe strain. Also, if there are other children they, too, can become resentful of all the attention that is being paid to their handicapped brother or sister. These situations need much thought and sensitive counselling to resolve.

Perhaps an even greater shock occurs when the baby appears to be perfect at birth, but in whom the genetic disorder only begins to show itself in the first few months or years of life. Hunter's syndrome is an example of this, the baby being normal at birth, but in whom physical and mental deterioration starts to arise at around 18 months to two years of age. Diagnosis will serve to confirm fears of an inherited disorder. Parents then will go through similar grief reactions as did other parents who have a child with a genetic disorder which is obvious at birth, such as Down's syndrome, or Apert's syndrome, for example.

Genetic disorders can also generate a good deal of guilty feelings in the parents. They feel that it is their fault that their child has been born with the particular syndrome. Again, explanation of the ways of genetic inheritance can help to overcome some of these feelings.

The wider family, not to mention close friends (who may also be in the reproductive years themselves) will be affected by the birth, or subsequent development of, a handicapped child. Parents who have accurate knowledge of their baby's condition will be in a better position to answer queries as to what is wrong with their baby, and how it will affect the life of the family in the future.

A handicapped child can bring families closer together in their support for the parents and the care of the child. Friends, too, will often rally round and give practical help and moral support. But occasionally the opposite reaction is uppermost and contact with parents and their baby ceases abruptly. With a handicapped child, one learns quickly who is a friend!

Life is never the same after the birth of any baby. With the birth of a handicapped baby, this change is increased a hundredfold. Hospital and clinic visits will need to be fitted into the daily round, special treatments or foods may need to be given or in-patient spells may be necessary. And all this on top of caring for a physically and/or mentally handicapped child who is not developing along the same lines as everyone else's baby. No wonder parents became quite exhausted, particularly as normal sleep patterns in the baby may be difficult to establish. Help from a variety of agencies should be made available to parents who have a baby suffering under these, and similar, conditions.

Accurate **diagnosis** is one of the most important first-line aspects. Following on from this, information can then be given as to what the future holds. This can take up much time, as parents will need to go away to think about the implications for their future lives. During this time many potential day-to-day problems will occur to them. So, once again, an important part of helping parents to come to terms with their baby's handicap is allowing time – maybe again and again – for discussion. Worries and fears need to be voiced so that explanations can be given, together with information on various agencies that can offer practical help.

Social workers will need to be involved with the family from the early days. Advice on help available, be it financial or local respite care facilities, for example, can do much to relieve the isolation felt by parents.

Respite care facilities will become more necessary as time goes by. Here families, closely vetted for suitability, volunteer to look after a handicapped child in their own home for a given period of time. This may be for a weekend only, or for a two-week break. This allows the parents of the handicapped child – and also any other children in the family – to go perhaps to a wedding or other family celebration or to enjoy a holiday without the continual worry of the care of a handicapped member. The 'host' family receive payment for their input into the care of the child. People who offer respite care facilities are frequently themselves working in the field of handicap, and so are well used to caring for handicapped children. Parents can thus be sure that their child is receiving the best possible care whilst they are away.

This brief break from the continual care can do much to relieve the exhaustion of the parents. Of importance is the chance for husband and wife to be together for some time to pursue common interests which are impossible to indulge with a handicapped child – for example, walking or a visit to the theatre. This aspect is probably of greater importance in today's society than a generation or two ago. Few parents today have the support of an extended family who will share the burden of care of children.

Self-help groups, of which a number have been formed over the past decade, certainly in the UK and USA, can also provide much support. It is good to be able to write, meet or telephone a family who have a child with a similar syndrome. Day-to-day management of problems can be talked over in an informal manner. Many of these self-help groups also provide useful material on the specific condition as well as arranging meetings for members. Many of these self-help groups are registered charities which organize fund-raising activities for research. These groups, together with social worker input, give valuable information regarding various items of equipment available for disabled living.

It is important that every handicapped child has his/her abilities, both physical and mental, assessed regularly on an ongoing basis. This can be done at a hospital, a clinic specializing in this purpose or at the child's own doctor's surgery if he is particularly interested in such problems.

Genetic counselling if the parents are contemplating a further pregnancy is important after the birth of a handicapped child. The exact diagnosis of the handicapping condition will need to be known, and a family tree of other possibly similarly handicapped members will need to be drawn up. There are a number of genetic counselling centres in the UK, if there is not one locally, where such advice can be given. (The addresses of these are given at the end of the book.) Any future pregnancy must be monitored carefully, with techniques such as ultrasonic scanning, chorionic villus sampling and amniocentesis.

Finally, **bereavement counselling** may be necessary at a later date. Many children with specific handicapping conditions cannot look forward to a normal life span. Death, in a number of syndromes, can occur in the late teenage years or early twenties. Even though they have been led to expect this, the actual event is a shattering blow to parents. From a busy life caring for their handicapped child, suddenly the days seem long and empty. Feelings of relief are mixed with the inevitable feelings of sadness and loss. This again can lead to an excess of the guilt normally felt after a death: 'Perhaps there could have been more done for our child?' 'Perhaps we were not as dedicated as we should have been?' And most pertinent of all in a genetically acquired condition, 'Was it our fault?' Parents will need much sympathetic support over the weeks and months following the death of a handicapped child.

All is not gloom, however, following the birth of a child with an inherited handicap. Families can be brought closer together in the care of their child. Pleasure can also result from helping with the everyday successes of life with a handicap. Many families will be certain that their quality of life is enhanced by their handicapped child with his/her own unique personality.

As our knowledge of the causes and effects of handicap increases, the more help will be given to members of our society – all over the world.

Achondroplasia

Alternative name

Chondro-dystrophy.

Incidence

The incidence of achondroplasia is thought to be around one in every 25 000 births. There are between 25 and 30 babies born with achondroplasia each year in the UK. The mode of inheritance would suggest this figure is variable, due to the inability to predict new mutations, which can also result in achondroplasia. Both sexes can be affected, and it is possible to diagnose achondroplasia at birth. A number of achondroplastic pregnancies are known to miscarry, or the baby dies in the early weeks of life, particularly if the birth has been premature.

History

There are quite a large number of conditions and syndromes in which short stature is a prominent feature. Achondroplasia is unique in that the limbs are short, whilst the trunk is of a normal size. This is obvious at birth. The short stature of other conditions will only become obvious as the child matures.

Many achondroplastic men and women used to be the 'small people' working in circuses. This was the only occupation open to them until comparatively recently when enlightenment regarding suitable careers became the norm. Achondroplasia is now no bar to many jobs and professions, including medicine and teaching.

Causation

The mode of inheritance is twofold. Achondroplasia can be inherited as an autosomal dominant characteristic or can arise as a new mutation. It is thought that the latter accounts for most of the babies born with achondroplasia. It has been suggested that advanced paternal age may be a factor, but this has not been proved. The basic fault is that the epiphyseal plates of the limbs fail to produce adequate cartilage tissue. This starts before birth.

Characteristics

Skeletal effects
Short stature: this is of a very particular type. The arms and legs are short, whilst the trunk and head are of normal size. Specialist charts are currently being produced to monitor the growth of achondroplastic children. The usual charts will not give a true picture of whether the child is growing satisfactorily or not, due to the disproportion in the body configuration in an achondroplastic child.

Head size gives rise to the appearance of being out of proportion to the trunk. There are a number of reasons for this. Head circumference is on the upper limits of normal, and also achondroplastic children usually have a broad, prominent forehead with often a larger than normal lower jaw. The bridge of the nose is also often flattened, and this adds to the optical illusion of a top-heavy head. In contrast to this, the base of the skull and the foramen magnum are small. This latter fact can sometimes cause compression of the spinal cord in this region, giving rise to respiratory problems. Some achondroplastic children have died suddenly and unexpectedly from this cause. Hydrocephalus, due to the abnormalities of the foramen magnum at the base of the skull, occurs in a few children with achondroplasia. This, too, will add to the disproportionate size of the head.

The **pelvis**, if X-rays are taken, also has abnormal features. The roof of the hip-joint is flat with a protruding bony spike. This can account, in part, for the unusual waddling gait of many people with achondroplasia. The fact of having very short legs also makes for an unusual walking pattern – especially when trying to keep up with long-legged companions!

The normal curves of the **spine** are accentuated. The lower lumbar curve is more marked than usual. This has little effect during childhood, but can give rise to lower back pain later in life.

Eventual **height** rarely reaches more than 55 in (140 cm).

Hands are broad and short, the lack of length being in the shortness of the metacarpals (from wrist to knuckles). Fingers in contrast are of normal length. The achondroplastic child cannot close his fingers together; they remain widely spaced in spite of all his efforts to approximate them.

Children with achondroplasia are often **hypotonic**. Due to this, they are often late in sitting and starting to walk. It is inadvisable to put too much pressure on them to hurry these skills along, as the combination of weak muscles and a large head puts a great strain on the spine with the probable effect of increasing the lordosis in the lumbar region. **Mental abilities** fall within the normal range, and intellectual abilities can be high. Psychologically, most achondroplastic children are well adjusted to their small size. But occasionally problems with body image can occur.

Ears: frequent middle ear infections are common. Later a conductive deafness can occur, due to the repeated ear infections. Sensori-neural deafness can also occur.

Management implications

These revolve largely around the short stature and its associated problems.

Short stature: problems with this aspect of achondroplasia will increase as the child matures. During infancy and the toddler years, lack of height is not too noticeable, but around the early school years it becomes obvious when the achondroplastic child stands alongside his/her peers. Orthopaedic treatment to lengthen limbs has been available in recent years, and research into the effects of giving growth hormone at appropriate times during the growing years is proceeding.

Practical aids, such as suitable seating, low shelves for storage of personal possessions, smaller sports equipment and general low-level living devices can make the life of the achondroplastic child easier. From the teenage years on, difficulties with ticket machines, high steps onto buses and trains as well as driving problems – to mention just a few – must all be appreciated, and help given wherever possible.

Emotional effects, both on the affected child and the family, must not be forgotten. Parents of normal height can become greatly distressed by their child's difficulties, and where the inheritance is obvious, the parent also affected can suffer from guilt reactions. Sensitive counselling of the whole family, with time to think through all the implications of short stature in particular, should be available. Care must also be taken to ensure that the child with achondroplasia is not treated as younger than his/her chronological age. It is all too easy to forget that in all aspects of development, other than height, the child is exactly the same as his peers, with similar needs – and, of course, potentially with similar behaviour. (Clearly this applies equally to all children of short stature.)

Orthopaedic abnormalities can result from abnormalities in the spine. 'Slipped discs' in the lower lumbar region are not uncommon in later life, and must be appropriately treated, probably by surgery. Leg lengthening operations and operations to correct excessively bowed legs can be undertaken in selected cases, and will do much to improve the quality of life. Watch must be kept for spinal cord compression – weakness and tingling in lower limbs – due to the abnormality in the region of the foramen magnum. Most importantly, breathing patterns must be watched carefully during childhood.

Hearing: the frequent attacks of otitis media must be treated quickly and adequately. Hearing assessment following attacks of infection should also be carried out to determine if hearing has been affected by the infective process. Myringotomy may need to be performed to counteract conductive deafness.

The future

Sufferers from achondroplasia have a normal life span, and are generally healthy individuals, as long as spinal abnormalities are not severe. Symptoms of cord compression (for example, weakness, pain or tingling in arms or legs) must be investigated urgently and treated. Job prospects are limited only by the lack of inches, as intellectual ability should not be affected. But with recent advances, this aspect of life shows more promise.

Achondroplasia is no bar to conception and pregnancy, although the delivery of the baby will need to be by caesarian section due to the pelvic abnormalities in most cases. Genetic counselling is advisable before embarking on a planned pregnancy. There is a 50% chance of the condition being inherited if one parent is achondroplastic and a 75% chance if both parents have the bone disorder.

Self-help groups

Bone Dysplasia Group (part of Child Growth Foundation)
2 Mayfield Avenue
London W4 1PW
(Tel. 081 994 7625; 081 995 0257)

This is a network of families offering advice on problems associated with achondroplasia and other conditions with lack of normal bone growth.

Disabled Living Foundation
346 Kensington High Street
London W14 8NS

Equipment for the Disabled
2 Foredown Drive
Portslade
Sussex BW4 2BB

Aicardi's syndrome

Incidence

The incidence of Aicardi's syndrome is not known. But as the definitive triad of signs are recognized this syndrome may not be as rare as was originally supposed. Only girls are affected due to the mode of inheritance, and all races seem to be involved. Certain criteria for a diagnosis of Aicardi's syndrome have recently been described. Similar signs and symptoms occur in other conditions, and it is probable that these, at times, are confused with true Aicardi's syndrome sufferers.

History

In the late 1960s, Dr. Aicardi described in the French literature a recognizable set of signs and symptoms now known as Aicardi's syndrome. By 1980, over 100 patients had been identified. In 1982, the genetic basis for the syndrome was reported.

Causation

At the present state of knowledge, Aicardi's syndrome seems to arise due to chromosomal abnormality of the X chromosome. It is probable that most usually this abnormality occurs as a new mutation, as there has only been one reported family with two children with the same condition. Only girls are affected as the condition seems to be incompatible with life in the male foetus. At present, ante-natal diagnosis is not possible.

Characteristics

Infantile spasms are one of the invariable characteristics of Aicardi's syndrome. These are convulsions of a specific type which begin in early infancy. Many of these fits can occur during the course of the day, and are sometimes known as 'infantile spasms' or 'salaam attacks' due to the position taken by the baby during a convulsion – rather like a formal bow. 'Hypsarrhythmia' is a further name. This type of convulsion continues to occur in Aicardi's syndrome throughout life in a modified form. These continual fits are very damaging to brain function, occurring as they do with such frequency.

The EEG features of Aicardi's syndrome are unusual and quite unique. There is obvious independent activity of the two halves of the brain on the tracing. It has been suggested that this may be due, in part, to the absence, or gross abnormality, of a specific part of the brain – the corpus callosum.

Eye abnormalities: the whole eye is often small. But the particular abnormality of the eye in Aicardi's syndrome is the appearance of the retina. When viewed with an ophthalmoscope, a number of 'punched out' areas are seen in this vital part of the eye. With this appearance blindness would seem to be inevitable, but this is not always so, although vision must, of necessity, be restricted. Nevertheless, sufferers frequently do become blind as they get older.

Brain abnormalities can be seen on CT scanning and magnetic resonance imaging. Specific areas of the brain – the corpus callosum (that part of the brain linking the two cerebral hemispheres together) – are affected. This feature results in severe **developmental delay** and **mental retardation**. All aspects of development are affected, both large and fine movements as well as speech. The restricted vision also adds to the problems of fine movements.

These are the three major problem areas which are to be found in all sufferers from Aicardi's syndrome. Other abnormalities are also commonly seen, but are not always present.

The **spinal column** often shows fused vertebrae or only partially developed vertebrae. As a result of this **scoliosis** frequently occurs, giving rise to respiratory problems due to restricted breathing movements. This picture is made worse by ribs being often misshapen or sometimes absent altogether. So the whole function of the chest – both heart and lungs – is under stress.

Deformities of the **hands** can also be present. The size of the baby's **head** can be small, and does not show the usual continuing growth. So the head circumference (a routine measurement in all babies which is indicative of brain development) is frequently on the lower line of the centile charts.

Management implications

Convulsions: these are especially difficult to control. Some sufferers have had to be prescribed as many as seven different anti-convulsants to control the seizures. ACTH has been used to good effect, and particularly so when given in the early months. It is thought that early control of convulsions, as far as is possible, may help to reduce further brain dysfunction.

Visual problems: the exact extent of the visual loss is difficult to diagnose accurately, due both to the anatomical effects in the retina and to the mental handicap found in Aicardi's syndrome children. Little help can be given due to the patchy loss of retinal tissue – this latter being vital for normal vision.

Developmental delay and **mental retardation** are profound and will need full-time skilled help as the child matures. Few children with Aicardi's syndrome develop any speech. Walking is usually achieved, but can be very late in occurring. Self-help skills, such as feeding and dressing, will be only slowly, if ever, achieved. Schools for profoundly handicapped pupils will be necessary. Respite care in order that parents can have a break from caring for their handicapped child should be made available if at all possible. It is important that other children in the family should be able to have an active holiday without the restrictions necessary for the care of their handicapped brother or sister.

Children with Aicardi's syndrome do seem to be especially prone to coughs and colds. These infections can often extend to their lower respiratory tract giving rise to bronchitis or pneumonia. The relative immobility of the child is not helpful in preventing these complications.

The future

This is bleak for sufferers from Aicardi's syndrome. Full-time care will need to be given throughout life. Control of seizures will also be a life-long problem, and many children succumb to respiratory tract infections.

The description of Aicardi's syndrome being of such recent origin, there are no substantiated reports as to how long these children can be expected to live. The oldest known survivor was 15 years old in 1989.

Self-help group

Recently a self-help group, known as CORPAL, has been formed. This includes families with children who have agenesis of the corpus callosum with no additional problems. The effects of this latter disorder are very variable, ranging from completely normal development to severe handicap.

The address to contact is:

CORPAL
7 Bromley Avenue
Flixton
Manchester M31 3HV
(Tel. 061 748 0014)

Aims and provisions: support and information for families; international links; promotion of research.

Albinism

Incidence

Albinism is a rare condition. There are a number of variants in which individuals are affected differently. Many affected people have to lead an altered life-style due to their albinism. It is thought to occur in approximately one in 200 000 people overall. Albinism occurs in all races, being more common in some peoples than others. For example, the incidence in France is 1 in 100 000, whilst the incidence in the San Blas Indians of Panama is seven in 1000.

There are a number of other syndromes which have albinism as part of their characteristics.

History

Albinos, the name by which people with albinism are frequently known, have been recognized for centuries. The name was originally applied by the Portuguese to white African negroes.

The name is also applied to animals and plants lacking pigment.

Causation

Albinism is a genetically inherited disease, most forms being transmitted in an autosomal recessive manner. The basic fault is one of an inborn error of metabolism, the enzyme tyrosinase being defective. So melanin – the pigment giving eye, hair and skin colour – is not available. This is in spite of there being normal numbers of pigment-forming cells (melanocytes) in the basal layer of the skin. But due to defective tyrosinase activity, these cells are not able to produce melanin.

There are several different types of albinism, which can be difficult to distinguish clinically. In one type there may some pigmented naevi on the body, and the hair in coloured races may be yellow instead of white. This would suggest that in this particular type there is some tyrosinase activity.

Albinism may also be partial, so that the full effects of complete melanin lack are not seen. Very blonde children with fine, delicate skin which burns easily on exposure to the sun probably have a minimal form of albinism. A type of albinism can be part of the clinical pattern of two further syndromes – Waardenburg's syndrome, which is associated with deafness and Chediak–Higashi syndrome, which also has blood and immunological problems associated with the condition. Eyes alone can be affected – ocular albinism – and this type is thought to be inherited in an X-linked manner.

Ante-natal diagnosis is only possible by biopsy of the foetal skin, which is rarely done.

Characteristics

Skin: albinos have a very fair skin which, without the protection of the necessary melanin in the skin, burns very readily in sunlight. Along with this fair skin goes white, silky hair. Eyebrows, eyelashes and other body hair are also white.

Eyes: the iris is very pale, pink or blue in colour. The redness of the retina can sometimes be seen through this translucent iris. As a result of this, photophobia (dislike of light) is common. Abnormalities in the visual pathways are always present in true albinism. Defective ante-natal development of optic fibres and poor formation of part of the retina due to lack of pigment is the basic problem. This leads to much reduced vision. Nystagmus – rapid backwards and forwards movement of the eyes – can also be present. Strangely enough, nystagmus does not interfere too much with vision, although some children develop an unusual head posture in an effort to compensate for the flickering of their eyes. This nystagmus in those albinos who show it usually improves with advancing years. Squints can also be present, although not invariably so.

Management implications

Skin: very great care needs to be taken with albino children in sunlight. Even dull days, with the sun behind cloud, can cause burning if the skin is exposed. Cover-up clothes are essential at all times and adequate sun-screen creams are also advisable. In hot sunny countries the problems can be acute.

Eyes: vision must be checked on a regular basis, and corrective lenses prescribed as far as is possible. It is especially important that school-age children should receive yearly visual checks. Vision can deteriorate rapidly during periods of rapid growth in all children, and albino children are specially at risk. It is frequently not possible to obtain perfect vision, due to the eye developmental abnormality which is always present in complete albinism. Vision does not deteriorate with age. Dark glasses are often necessary to protect the eyes from light due to the lack of protective pigment in the iris. Squints, when present, should be corrected orthoptically or surgically so as to maximize on all possible vision. Early correction of squints is vital if amblyopia – lack of vision in one eye – is to be avoided.

Education: about 20% of albino children will need special educational facilities due to their visual problems. These children are not blind, although their vision is such as to come within the legal definition of blindness. Emphasis in schools should be put on those activities at which the children can do well. Other children, with fewer visual problems will be able to attend mainstream schools, but with care always being taken regarding their sensitive skins.

The future

Albinism does not restrict life span. However, career prospects can be limited. Work outside in all weathers has to be avoided due to the skin problems.

Restricted distance vision in many cases will give rise to problems of obtaining a driving licence. Near vision, however, is usually good, so careers needing fine, close work are most suitable, and especially as these kind of skills also involve inside work. In this way skin problems are avoided. Children with normally pigmented skin can be born to a couple who both have albinism. Genetic counselling should be given due to the number of variants of the condition. Careful scrutiny of family trees, ancestors with very pale skins and fair hair and maybe other abnormalities will give clues as to possible inheritance patterns.

Skin cancers can arise more readily due to the lack of protective melanin. So any patch of skin which shows signs of permanent reddening, soreness or excess itching should receive immediate attention.

Self-help group

Albino Fellowship
16 Neward Crescent
Ayr, Scotland KA7 4DS
(Tel. 0292 70336)

Aims and provisions: Support and fellowship; leaflets on special problems.

Albright's syndrome

Alternative names

Albright's hereditary osteodystrophy (AHO); pseudohypoparathyroidism.

Incidence

Albright's syndrome is a rare condition. The exact number of children affected is unknown, but nevertheless the condition is well-documented. Basically this syndrome arises from a fault in calcium and phosphate metabolism in the body which in turn is due to faulty parathyroid hormone activity.

Both boys and girls can be affected, but with girls more commonly seen with the syndrome.

The biochemical abnormality need not give rise to symptoms and can be found in totally asymptomatic and clinically normal people. The abnormality is only discovered when specific routine testing is undertaken in relatives of children who have Albright's syndrome.

History

In 1942 Albright first recognized the syndrome as being due to a failure of the action of the parathyroid hormone on calcium and phosphates in the body. Research continued, and eventually in 1980 the basic molecular defects of the disease were described.

Causation

Albright's syndrome is a genetic disorder with some uncertainties still existing as to the exact mode of inheritance. It may be that the syndrome is X-linked, which would account for the higher incidence in girls. However, other authorities consider Aicardi's syndrome to be inherited as an autosomal dominant characteristic, but with sex modifications.

Characteristics

Albright's syndrome may not be recognized until mid-childhood, although convulsions due to the altered calcium and phosphate levels can occur in infancy, when the diagnosis can be made.

The following characteristics are found in the complete syndrome in mid-childhood.

Short stature: this is not usually as marked as in many other syndromes (cf. Turner's syndrome). Body proportions are normal with legs and arms in keeping with the rest of the body (cf. achondroplasia) Most people with Albright's syndrome reach a final height of around 5 ft, which is quite an acceptable height for most activities.

Obesity occurs commonly and makes the lack of inches appear more obvious. Typically, Albright's children have plump, round faces with a short neck. This tendency to excessive weight gain can also be noted before birth, so that many babies with Albright's syndrome have a high birth weight. Weight gain is also rapid in the first few months. (Whilst the above picture of height and weight is usual in Albright's syndrome, these measurements can be within the normal range.)

Skeletal system: due to the abnormalities in calcium and phosphate metabolism, unusual calcification can occur in parts of the skeleton. For example, hips and pelvis can have abnormal bony configurations as well as limb bones.

Short fourth and fifth fingers are a fairly constant finding and can help in confirming the diagnosis. The shortness of these fingers is very specific, and is due to the relative shortness of the terminal phalanges of these digits.

Eyes: cataracts can occur in Albright's syndrome, although this is not an invariable finding.

Mental retardation: intelligence is sometimes normal in children with Albright's syndrome but the usual range of intelligence quotient is between 20 and 99, with a mean level of 60. The level of intelligence would seem to depend upon blood levels of calcium and phosphate. Those children with low levels are more likely to have a degree of retardation than those with normal levels of these chemicals.

Thyroid underactivity is more commonly found in children with Albright's syndrome than in the general population. It is important that this is diagnosed early if present, so that treatment with thyroid hormone can be given. It is thought probable that early treatment of this problem reduces the incidence of possible mental retardation.

Management implications

Hypocalcaemia: if low levels of blood calcium are found, treatment with vitamin D has been found to be effective. Calcium supplements may also be necessary, as may other drugs to reduce the amount of calcium excreted.

Hypothyroidism must be treated with replacement thyroid hormone if levels of this hormone are found to be low. Signs of hypothyroidism, such as weight gain, slow speech, a hoarse voice, scanty hair and dry skin should be watched for in a child known to have Albright's syndrome. Blood levels can then confirm the clinical diagnosis.

Dietary measures to reduce obesity should be undertaken (and kept up!). The help of a dietician should be enlisted as it is important that nutrition is adequate for proper growth and development. Dieticians, too, have a wealth of skills which make eating the right foods fun rather than restrictive. Over-weight children can suffer miseries at school. As well as being the target for teasing, they find it difficult to join in physical activities, and are often the last person to be asked to join a team. From the health point of view, excess weight puts unwanted strain on growing joints. There may also be a link with hypertension in later life. So all efforts should be made to keep weight gain to a minimum.

Mental retardation, if present, may need special schooling and extra help later in childhood. Routine developmental checks and, later, school performance tests, will determine if there are any problems. Children of normal intelligence with Albright's syndrome are perfectly able to cope with mainstream schooling. Care must be taken, however, that dietary regimes and any necessary medication are strictly controlled.

Eyes: cataracts will need ophthalmic assessment and treatment if present. Routine visual tests should be done to pick up problems early. Good lighting and some form of magnification can be helpful before any necessary operative procedures are undertaken.

Genetic counselling needs to be available when the reproductive years are reached.

The future

A normal life span is to be expected in adults with Albright's syndrome. However, watch should be kept on blood-pressure during adult years as severe hypertension is found in over half of the adults with this condition. This finding can predispose to early 'strokes' and/or coronary thrombosis. So treatment should be given to maintain blood pressure within normal limits as far as possible. Weight control will lessen the risks of hypertension.

Self-help group

None specific, but support and information on facilities available from:

Research Trust for Metabolic Diseases in Children (RTMDC)
53 Beam Street
Nantwich
Cheshire CW5 2NF
(Tel. 0270 629782)

Angelman's syndrome

Alternative name

Hitherto known as the 'happy puppet' syndrome.

Incidence

The exact number of children with Angelman's syndrome is not known, but over 80 definite cases have been reported in the literature.

History

Children with Angelman's syndrome were previously referred to as suffering from the 'happy puppet' syndrome, due to the rather jerky movements seen in association with outbursts of laughter. This name has now been dropped since more knowledge has been gained regarding the genetic basis for this condition.

Causation

Angelman's syndrome is a chromosomal disorder, the faulty chromosome being chromosome 15. There has been found to be a deletion in the same region of this chromosome as is seen in Prader–Willi syndrome. In spite of this, the two syndromes are very different clinically. It is thought that the problem in the case of Angelman's syndrome is derived from the maternal side, in distinction from Prader–Willi syndrome in which the defect is considered to arise from the father. Most children with this syndrome occur out of the blue, although five families have been reported to have two children with the same condition.

Angelman's syndrome is not evident at birth, but becomes obvious as the child matures. There is no ante-natal test available at present. It is advisable, if possible, that parents should receive genetic counselling before embarking upon a further pregnancy.

Characteristics

Microcephaly: at birth, the baby's head circumference is within normal limits. As the child grows, this important measurement is seen to fall behind the other parameters of growth, never reaching the normal size.

During infancy, **feeding** can be a problem, largely due to poor brain development, and so difficulties in sucking.

Normal **sleep patterns** are also often difficult to establish. Babies with Angelman's syndrome are frequently hyperactive, and seem to need little sleep – and that little at inappropriate times!

Developmental delay leading to severe **mental retardation** occurs over the early years. Babies up to approximately one year of age can appear to be progressing normally, but from then on, signs of delayed development are to be seen, in particular the following:

1. **Speech** is affected to a disproportionate degree. Expressive speech is never properly attained, although receptive language develops so that children with Angelman's syndrome are able to understand simple commands.
2. **Walking** is late, and a typical jerky gait in noticeable in the early years, although this does tend to improve in later childhood. Occasionally, the unusual gait produces deformities in joints, which may need correction at a later date.
3. **Arm movements** are also jerky and stereotyped. (These movements, combined with the unusual gait, gave rise to the name 'happy puppet'.)
4. **Hand flapping**, often associated with outbursts of **inappropriate laughter** is another obvious characteristic. The laughter is not thought to be connected with epilepsy – as can be the case – but rather due to involuntary motor activity.

Seizures are common during infancy and childhood and a characteristic pattern is seen on EEG tracing. These fits may decrease spontaneously in later life.

Facial features: children with Angelman's syndrome tend to have large mouths with widely spaced teeth. Tongues tend to protrude, and this is especially noticeable during the outbursts of laughter.

Children with Angelman's syndrome are usually happy and affectionate young people. One of the greatest problems associated with this syndrome is the child's inability to speak. But in spite of this handicap, children appear to enjoy life.

Management implications

Early **feeding** and **sleep** problems, with a varying degree of **hyperactivity**, will need help. Small, frequent feeds and a regular routine in an attempt to rationalize the sleeping pattern is the best method of approach. This can take much patience and support. Short-term sedation may be necessary to break the difficult sleeping pattern, and also to allow the parents to get some sleep themselves.

Speech therapy help is indicated as the speech problems become obvious. Non-verbal techniques of communication such as sign-language training may help to relieve some of the frustration felt by the child due to the lack of usual communication skills. It is rare that any understandable speech is ever attained.

Seizures will need to be controlled with anti-convulsants. Dosage and type of anti-convulsant will need to be checked on a regular basis as fits tend to reduce naturally later in childhood.

Mental retardation will require educational facilities for severely handicapped pupils, where there is an emphasis on training in self-help skills. This training will need to be continued in a suitable environment after statutory school-age has been passed.

The future

Regrettably, children with Angelman's syndrome will never be able to lead an independent life. Full-time care will be necessary, preferably in a warm, loving environment where some degree of suitable communication can take place.

Life expectancy is thought to be normal. There have been no reported children being born to sufferers from Angelman's syndrome.

Self-help group

Angelman Syndrome Support Group
15 Place Crescent
Waterlooville, Portsmouth
Hampshire PO7 5UR
(Tel. 0705 264224)

Apert's syndrome

Alternative names

Acrocephalo-syndactyly type 1; Vogt cephalo-syndactyly.

Incidence

Apert's syndrome is one of a group of syndromes which are characterized by premature fusion of the bones of the skull, together with malformations of the hands and feet. This type of acrocephalo-syndactyly is one of the most serious of the group.

The condition is rare, only occurring in between one in 100 000 to one in 160 000 births.

Both boys and girls can be affected, and the condition can be diagnosed at birth.

Causation

Apert's syndrome can be inherited as autosomal dominant. But few cases of direct inheritance from either parent are known. Most of the cases seem to arise as new mutations.

There have been suggestions that older fathers may be more at risk of having a child with Apert's syndrome, but this has not been conclusively proved.

Characteristics

The bones of the skull in new-born babies are normally separated from each other. This aids the process of birth by the skull being able to mould to the birth canal. Soon after birth the edges of these flat bones become joined together by fibrous tissue in specific places. These positions of fusion are known as the 'sutures' of the skull. It is at these positions that future skull growth occurs to accommodate the underlying growing brain. In Apert's syndrome (and also in other syndromes of a similar nature) these sutures fuse together prematurely. It is this early fusion that gives rise to the typical characteristics of the head and the face seen in children with this syndrome.

Head: the most striking features of babies born with Apert's syndrome is their high, prominent forehead, often with a marked swelling in the mid-line. The backs of the heads of these babies also tend to be more flattened than is usual.

Facial features: in contrast to the prominent forehead – and also often large lower jaw, noses are small and flattened. This can give rise to both breathing and feeding difficulties in the neo-natal period. **Eyes** are also large and prominent, and are usually widely set apart.

Ears tend to be low-set and a congenital hearing loss is frequently present.

The **hands** of babies with Apert's syndrome can also be malformed. The severity of this deformity can vary a good deal. Sometimes only webbing of the skin between the fingers is present, but the worst cases show some bones of the hands completely fused together, usually involving the second, third and fourth fingers. If this occurs the hands have a claw-like appearance.

Feet are usually normal, but in rare cases can have a similar appearance to the hands.

Mild **mental retardation** occurs in around 50% of children with Apert's syndrome – the remaining 50% having normal intelligence. Any slowing of abilities will gradually become apparent over the months and years, and will be picked up during routine developmental checks.

Hydrocephalus, caused by faulty drainage of cerebro-spinal fluid in the ventricles of the brain, is a not infrequent complication of Apert's syndrome.

A further unusual complication, seen in a large number of young people with this syndrome, is severe **acne** during the adolescent years.

Management implications

Initially, **feeding** and **breathing** difficulties commonly occur. The nasal abnormalities make it difficult, if not impossible, for the baby to breathe whilst he/she is feeding. So in the early days, nasogastric feeding will probably be necessary. By three to four months these problems resolve themselves as the nasal passages enlarge with general growth.

If **hydrocephalus** occurs, a 'shunt' will need to be inserted to drain the excess fluid away from the brain. This complication, so often seen in Apert's syndrome babies, can be difficult to diagnose in the early stages, as the more usual signs of hydrocephalus tend to be obscured by the unusual shape of the skull. Careful checks on neurological signs, such as increased tone in the lower limbs for example, and developmental patterns will be necessary to exclude this added problem.

Surgery to correct the premature fusion of the bones of the skull will need to be undertaken, and this may well mean a series of operations over the years. It is thought that these corrective procedures may help to prevent mental retardation. Surgery may also be necessary on hands, and sometimes feet, to achieve maximum function, and for cosmetic reasons.

Regular **developmental checks** are of vital importance to diagnose early any slowing, or regression, of physical function and other skills.

Due to frequent stays in hospital for various necessary operative procedures, Apert's syndrome children will need extra loving stimulation between these visits so that vital learning processes are not missed out.

Understanding and support for parents and child will need to be available, due not least to the unusual facial and limb features. Other children – and regrettably also adults – can be particularly unkind to children who look 'different'.

The future

Life expectancy for people with Apert's syndrome can be normal, but is dependent upon the degree of involvement of the central nervous system.

Career prospects are limited by the degree of disability experienced due to hand deformities, and also to mental abilities. Unusual facial features also make for some restrictions in work possibilities.

Self-help group

There is no specific Apert's syndrome group, but support, advice and friendship can be obtained from:

'Let's Face It' (Network for the Facially Disfigured)
10 Wood End
Crowthorne
Berks RG11 6DG

This organization, which has international links, has a junior branch linking parents who have facially disfigured children.

Arthrogryposis

Incidence

There are a number of similar conditions which all fall under the main heading of the arthrogryposes. The full name of the commonest of these is arthrogryposis multiplex congenita (AMC). Probably the next commonest sub-group is 'distal arthrogryposis' in which only the hands and feet are affected. There are a number of other variants described, all of which have similar characteristics, but show some specific features. For example, in some children there is more emphasis on weakness of the muscles, whilst others have greater problems with neurological involvement of certain spinal cord segments.

The incidence of the commonest sub-group – AMC – is around one baby in every 10 000 being born with the condition. Both boys and girls are equally affected.

Causation

The arthrogryposes are genetically inherited conditions. With the wide variety of known types, the inheritance pattern cannot be generalized. Distal arthrogryposis is inherited as an autosomal dominant condition, whilst AMC is thought to arise spontaneously as a new mutation. So it is important that when genetic counselling is given the exact diagnosis is known. In this way predictions of further children being born with the abnormality can be given more accurately.

Babies with arthrogryposis can be diagnosed at birth. Hints that foetal movements may be diminished can be confirmed by ultra-sound investigations over a specific period of time, for example one hour. Delivery can sometimes be difficult due to the relative immobility of the baby due to his genetic inheritance. This traumatic delivery can, at times, lead to some degree of mental handicap.

Characteristics

The common feature that affects children with any of the arthrogryposes is **joint deformities**. It is usual that many joints are affected. In distal arthrogryposis it is only the joints of the lower legs and forearms that are affected. All of these deformities are due to the soft tissues around the joints being contracted, or stiffened. Due to this, the joints themselves are rendered almost immobile, and certainly without normal, useful function.

The following description is of a baby born with the severe form of the commonest of the arthrogryposes – AMC.

Joint deformities: the baby with this form of arthrogryposis will lie in a very typical position soon after birth due to the deformities to be found in his/her joints. Shoulders will be pushed forward as arms are rotated inwards with flexed wrists and fingers turned into the palms of the hands. In a similar way feet are flexed into a position having the appearance of a 'club foot' deformity.

Muscles in many cases are small and weak, often being replaced by fibrous or fatty tissue. Without adequate muscle power, joints are made even more immobile. A very noticeable feature in some babies with AMC is the lack of normal elbow and/or knee creases, which is such as obvious feature of most new-born babies. This is directly due to the lack of muscle development.

Short stature can be a feature in later life, as normal growth of bone is, in part, dependent on adequate movement. Without normal muscle this is impossible. The shortness is not extreme, but nevertheless obvious.

Naevi: these 'strawberry' marks are very commonly seen in babies with AMC, and especially in the mid-line of the face and the body in general.

Following on from these minor abnormalities in the mid-line of the body can be the more serious ones of **defects in the abdominal wall**; **inguinal hernia**; **asymmetry of the face**. These problems fortunately only occur in relatively few babies with AMC.

Management implications

It is important that the diagnosis of arthrogryposis is made early on in the baby's life so that treatment to mobilize limbs, as far as possible, is started early.

Physiotherapy is the mainstay of treatment, and concentrates mainly on mobilizing any muscle tissue that is present. Passive stretching of affected limbs, with joints put gently through the full range of movement, on a regular basis, is of great value.

Splinting of affected joints in optimum position is also necessary. This has to be done very carefully in order to avoid damage to the weakened muscular tissue. The advice of an orthopaedic surgeon, working in close liaison with the physiotherapist, is vital to the future maximum function. Maximum mobility should be the aim, so that bone growth is diminished as little as possible.

Most children with arthrogryposis manage quite adequately in mainstream **schooling**. Stairs can be a problem, and adaptation with ramps, for example, may be necessary if buildings are not all on one level. Physical education lessons will not be possible for all but the most minimally affected children. Other suitable activities should be arranged during these lessons for the child with arthrogryposis if full integration into mainstream schooling is to be achieved. The help of the occupational therapy department can do much to give advice on suitable occupations, which can also help with limb mobility.

The future

Children with arthrogryposis can lead full, satisfying lives within the bounds of their physical limitations. Mental ability is not affected in any way by the condition, so any number of careers are open. Obviously those activities needing physical strength or mobility are not possible, but numerous other sedentary and intellectual pursuits are options.

Expected life span is not decreased by arthrogryposis.

Self-help group

The Arthrogryposis Group (TAG)
1 The Oaks
Gillingham
Dorset SP8 4SW
(Tel. 0747 822655)

Aims and provisions: support and information for affected families; research programmes; social events and annual conference; video available.

Asperger's syndrome

Incidence

The incidence of Asperger's syndrome is not yet known, as no large-scale detailed studies have been carried out, although research is continuing in this direction. Latest work seems to suggest that boys are affected around seven times more frequently than girls. This syndrome is generally referred to as occurring in those children who are amongst the more able of those suffering from autism. The classification is somewhat confused, but at the present time Asperger's syndrome refers to children with less severe autistic features. They are children who can use non-emotional speech, but who show obsessional interests and tend to be clumsy. The incidence of autism is thought to be around one in every 2500 live births, so Asperger's syndrome is but a part of this overall incidence.

History

It was in 1944 that an Austrian psychiatrist, Hans Asperger, first described the characteristics of children who showed lack of social adjustment and much self-absorption. Dr. Kanner, at much the same time, also reported similar features but with more emphasis on the specific speech and language problems. Dr. Lorna Wing in the UK has done much work on autism.

Causation

There is no known definitive cause of autism, or of Asperger's syndrome. Other syndromes, such as the fragile X syndrome, can all show autistic features to a greater or lesser degree. Dr. Asperger considered that this syndrome must be genetically transmitted. He noted a higher incidence of similar characteristics in the fathers of those children with the syndrome. Some children – about half of one series – had some history of birth problems, leading to the conclusion that in some cases organic brain deficiencies may be a causative factor.

Characteristics

In a recent seminar six features were noted to be present in sufferers from Asperger's syndrome.

1. Grave difficulties with **interactive play** with peers. Children with Asperger's syndrome do not wish to socialize and are unable to form

relationships with other children. They are seen as 'cold', 'immature' or 'eccentric', and so are usually left to play on their own.

2. Children with Asperger's syndrome become **totally absorbed** in one specific hobby or aspect of life, to the exclusion of every other facet of daily living. This interest may be anything from chess to stamp-collecting or astronomy, the subject often having a highly intellectual content.

3. Children with this syndrome need to adhere strictly to **routine** in all aspects of daily living. They become extremely upset if this stereotype is upset. For example, if on holiday the usual bedtime is relaxed this one minor alteration in the timetable can be very distressing for all the family!

4. **Speech and language** are often stereotyped, with a flat, monotonous, often expressively perfect, delivery. Comprehension of language appears to fall behind the normal expressive component. For example, jokes are often taken at their face value – with sometimes embarrassing consequences.

5. The vast majority of children with Asperger's syndrome show varying degrees of **clumsiness**. Actions are stiff, and often odd postures are taken up.

6. **Facial expression and gesture** used in association with speech is frequently inappropriate or clumsy. For example, yawning or smiling at the wrong time during a conversation is typical of the child with this syndrome.

These features are, of course, very similar to those of autism with which Asperger's syndrome is closely linked.

Management implications

It has been noted that the more able person with autism – Asperger's syndrome – usually shows an improvement with time. After the turmoils of adolescence are over, behaviour becomes more normal and acceptable. This may be due to care and teaching in specific areas, which is of great importance in children with Asperger's syndrome.

Social and communication skills: it is in this area of development that the most difficulties are experienced. Specific efforts need to be made to teach these skills, many of which are picked up automatically by the normal child. Normal social interaction is a closed book to most children with Asperger's syndrome. The normal give-and-take of socializing can be totally bemusing so that each set of situations with the appropriate response will have to be learned. This is quite possible to achieve given the liking for rote learning and stereotyped behaviour characteristic of the child with Asperger's syndrome. It is important that the child is not allowed to withdraw into himself to avoid social activities. This is counter-productive, but a very understandable way of avoiding difficult situations.

Language may be delayed and speech therapists can pinpoint the specific areas of difficulty. For example, words which are used to describe actions (verbs) are more of a mystery than words used to denote objects (nouns). It is important that teaching of language will take place alongside the teaching of social skills in familiar situations. This will help comprehension and assist in preventing stereotypical and obsessive behaviour.

Behavioural therapy: dealing with the obsessive ritualistic behaviour of children with Asperger's syndrome is one of the more difficult problems. Probably the best approach is a graded change of behaviour patterns, starting off with small steps and continuing slowly until the rituals no longer obtrude in normal life.

Schooling: dealing with the disabling problems caused by Asperger's syndrome is complex, needing much sensitivity to help the sufferer. Specialists with a particular interest in the syndrome can be found by contacting the support group. There is no one particular type of school suitable for all Asperger's syndrome sufferers. Some children will be able to manage in mainstream schooling, whilst others may fare better in any one of a number of specialized schools. Each child needs to be placed according to their own specific abilities.

The future

Depending on the severity of the manifestation of Asperger's syndrome some form of employment is often possible in adult life. Work involving a regular routine is the best choice, and the sympathetic understanding of eccentricities by employers and fellow-workers is important. Other, more severely affected, men and women, particularly those with speech and language difficulties, are unable to hold down any kind of job, so sheltered accommodation and care will be needed for life. But, even in severely affected people, a reduction in disability does seem to occur with time.

Self-help group

Asperger Support Network is part of:

The National Autistic Society
276 Willesden Lane
London NW2 5RB
(Tel. 081 451 1114)

Aims and provisions: support and information; contact with local groups; schools and centres managed for adolescents and adults; courses and conferences; research activities.

Ataxia-telangiectasia

Alternative names

Louis–Barr syndrome; Boder–Sedgwick syndrome.

Incidence

Ataxia-telangiectasia is a very rare condition, affecting only between one baby in every 30 000 to 50 000. There are a comparatively high number of cases in some countries, Turkey being quoted as one of these. This is possibly due to the fact that intermarriage between close relatives is more common. Both boys and girls can be equally affected.

Causation

Ataxia-telangiectasia is thought to be transmitted as an autosomal recessive characteristic. This would account for the high incidence in countries where it is more likely that parents are related. There may be further cases where there is no direct link, the condition being due to a new mutation. Recently gene mapping has demonstrated that the ataxia-telangiectasia is located on chromosome 11.

Ante-natal testing is difficult at present, and modes of inheritance strongly depends on looking at other members of the family in detail. Serum alpha-fetoprotein levels are frequently raised in people with ataxia-telangiectasia, but not invariably so. This fact can help with diagnosis.

Ataxia-telangiectasia is not apparent at birth and only becomes obvious between the ages of one and two, when the child starts to walk.

Characteristics

Walking: As soon as a definite walking pattern is established it is noticeable that the toddler is more unsteady on his/her feet than would be expected at the developmental stage reached. This is quite apparent after the age when tumbles are the norm for the new walker. This ataxia persists throughout life and, regrettably, tends to worsen as the child matures. Later, involuntary movements of limbs become apparent, much as seen in certain types of cerebral palsy. (In ataxia-telangiectasia the basic pathology is a very much reduced number of specialized (Purkinje) cells in the cerebellum; that part of the brain associated with the control of balance. As with many disorders there may be an enzyme defect involved.)

Speech can become slurred and disjointed, again due to the difficulty of control of muscular movement. But after the initial period of deterioration in the pre-school years, this particular problem should stabilize, and the child with ataxia-telangiectasia can always make him/herself understood.

Prominent blood-vessels – **telangiectases** – appear later on the white part of the eyes. Little dilated vessels are seen to be coursing over the eye, rather as if the child had conjunctivitis without the surrounding inflammation seen in this infective condition. Unlike conjunctivitis the eyes are not sore or itchy. These characteristic changes in the eye can also sometimes be seen on the ears.

Infections of all kinds are frequent and even minor ones can be serious. This is due to an associated defect in the immune system of the child with ataxia-telangiectasia. Respiratory infections, which can be difficult to treat adequately, are the most common.

Malignancies, at any site in the body, are more common than usual. It is thought that around one-third of all ataxia-telangiectasia sufferers will develop cancer at some time in their lives.

Sensitivity to radiation is a further feature of ataxia-telangiectasia. This becomes of vital importance when radiation is needed to treat any cancerous growths that occur. Fibrous tissue, as a result of scarring due to the radiation, almost always results even with the carefully controlled doses given to treat malignant growths. (Normal X-ray examination – for example, necessary to diagnose the exact nature of a respiratory infection – is not harmful, the dosage being low.)

Slowing of **growth** can occur in some children with ataxia-telangiectasia, but this does not always occur.

Sexual maturity is often late in being attained. This is due, in girls, to lack of ovarian growth and so of function.

Management implications

Although there is no specific treatment which can halt the course of the disease, there is much that can be done to make life easier for ataxia-telangiectasia sufferers and their families.

The **ataxia** can occasionally be helped by the giving of anti-spasmodic drugs. But the ongoing nature of the situation must eventually be appreciated, and a suitable life-style organized.

Most children will be confined to a wheelchair by the time they are ten years old, and schooling has to be geared to this. A school for physically handicapped pupils may be needed if buildings in local mainstream schools are not suitable – for example, lack of ramps and suitable toileting facilities.

Typewriters or wordprocessors are useful if the ataxia affects hands and arms, making writing illegible. Special guards can be fitted making it easier for the child to hit the correct keys.

Infections must be reduced to a minimum as far as is possible. For example, relatives and friends should be asked to stay away from the child if they think they are incubating a respiratory tract infection. It is a practical impossibility to avoid all infection in children, but these must be treated quickly and adequately by the appropriate antibiotic.

The early stages of **cancer** must be watched for, and any suspicious symptoms investigated fully and quickly. In particular, any low-grade fever continuing for any length of time must be viewed seriously. This may be due to a hidden source of infection or early manifestation of cancerous growth. Following on from this, special care with radiation therapy must be taken if cancer does occur, due to the high sensitivity of ataxia-telangiectasia sufferers to this form of treatment.

The future

Life expectancy for the child with ataxia-telangiectasia is not great, and many will die in their twenties or thirties. Overwhelming infection or the results of malignant disease account for most of these tragically early deaths.

Self-help group

Ataxia-telangiectasia Society
42 Parkside Gardens
Wollaton
Nottingham NG8 2PQ
(Tel. 0602 287025)

Aims and provisions: support and contact with families; information by leaflet and meetings.

Batten's disease

Alternative names

Batten–Vogt syndrome; Kufs' disease (adult form).

Incidence

Batten's disease is one of a wide group of diseases which have a metabolic basis for the signs and symptoms seen. There are over 1000 of these metabolic conditions described. They all have in common some enzyme malfunction which results in imbalances of chemicals in the body. Signs and symptoms will be wide-ranging depending on which system of the body is most involved. The substances involved in Batten's disease (and related conditions) are the neuronal ceroid-lipo-fuscinoses (NCL). Batten's disease has at least four main types, the age of onset of the symptoms being the main differentiating point. It is a comparatively rare condition, although an incidence of one in 13 000 of the infantile type has been reported from Finland. Both boys and girls can be equally affected.

History

Many of the metabolic disorders have been known and described for years. It is only fairly recently, however, that the biochemical basis for many of these conditions has been understood. With increasing knowledge more groups of signs and symptoms (syndromes!) are being found to be due to an enzyme malfunction.

Causation

Batten's disease is inherited as an autosomal recessive characteristic. The gene is located on chromosome 16, and ante-natal diagnosis has been possible by amniocentesis. Genetic counselling for future pregnancies is advisable.

Characteristics

The four different types of Batten's disease are all characterized by progressive mental and physical deterioration, loss of vision and convulsions. Each of these aspects has a different emphasis in the different types.

Infantile type (also known as the Santavouri or Finnish type)
This type becomes obvious at around one year of age. **Convulsions** occur at this time and a fall-off in **mental development** is noticed. The normal development abilities slow, and the 'milestones', tested by routine developmental checks, fall behind the norm. The ability to walk, instead of gradually increasing in strength and stability, becomes more and·more unsteady.

Head circumference (that excellent indicator of brain growth in the early years) fails to increase along the normal growth lines as plotted on growth charts, and microcephaly becomes obvious within a year or two.

Regrettably the course of the disease is rapidly downhill, and death usually occurs between the ages of five and six years, most often due to some intercurrent infection.

Late infantile type (also known as Jansky–Bielchowsky type)
Development proceeds normally until two to four years of age. At around this time, **convulsions** occur, which become more and more difficult to control.

The child's **walking** becomes increasingly clumsy and ataxic, and fine motor movements are also affected. Many of the skills already learned in both these areas of development become increasingly difficult to perform.

Along with these problems goes an increasing **visual loss**. This is due to a degeneration of the retina, again as a direct result of the enzyme defect. Nothing can be done to halt this process, and the child will eventually lose most of his/her vision.

Mental deterioration also occurs, and skills previously learned are lost.

As with the infantile form, death occurs in childhood, usually by ten years of age, and, again, an intercurrent infection is the commonest cause.

Juvenile NCL (also known as Speilmeyer–Vogt disease)
This type does not make its presence known until between six and ten years of age. The first signs of this form of Batten's disease is a diminution in vision. This is due to changes in the pigment of the retina. As a result of this the ability to transmit images to the brain is lost.

Within a few months of this deterioration, there is a slowing of **mental abilities**. **Convulsions** also occur as with the other forms of Batten's disease with an earlier onset.

Again, muscular co-ordination problems occur, and **walking** becomes ataxic and fine hand movements become clumsy and difficult to perform.

avoided as far as is possible. This, of course, is incredibly difficult to avoid in the rough and tumble of childhood. But preventative measures such as protective padding or clothing over bony prominences, such as elbows and knees, can avoid at least some of the injury. Sympathetic handling is often needed to persuade the child with Ehlers–Danlos syndrome to wear such protective clothing. If injury to the skin does occur which needs stitching, closure of the wound with tape is the preferred method of treatment. Routine stitching can give rise to further problems with healing. If surgery for any reason has to be undertaken, particular care will be needed to be sure that adequate healing takes place.

Teeth: meticulous and ongoing dental care is vital for children and adults with Ehlers–Danlos syndrome. The probable early loss of teeth with some types makes good fitting and maintenance of dentures a priority.

Eyes: retinal detachment must be suspected and excluded if there is any sudden loss of vision.

The future

Children with Ehlers–Danlos syndrome will need to be protected, as far as possible without compromising their spontaneous energies, from injury. This will need the sympathetic cooperation of playmates as well as knowledge and understanding of their condition by teaching staff. Careers advice will need to be geared towards more sedentary occupations.

Pregnancy can often result in premature birth due to early rupture of the membranes which, at this time, are also involved in the general connective tissue abnormality.

Life expectancy is normal in Ehlers–Danlos syndrome with the exception of the type in which there is particular fragility of the large blood vessels. Here, rupture can lead to a fatal outcome.

Self-help group

Ehlers–Danlos Support Group
2 High Grath
Richmond
North Yorkshire DL10 4DG
(Tel. 0344 57695)

Aims and provisions: mutual support of affected families by telephone and letter; information about condition – leaflets and tapes; list of specialists with particular interest in condition.

Epidermolysis bullosa

Alternative names

There are a number of sub-types of this condition, for example epidermolysis bullosa Mendes da Costa and epidermolysis bullosa Koebner type, but all have the prefix 'epidermolysis bullosa' or EBS.

Incidence

The true incidence of epidermolysis bullosa is not entirely clear. In the USA a specific number of large families have been documented, many of whom have the condition. From these studies it is estimated that there are at least 50 000 Americans – mainly children – suffering from epidermolysis bullosa. It is thought that there are around 2500 sufferers in the UK.

Causation

EBS is inherited as an autosomal dominant except for the two sub-types EBS lethal type, which is inherited in an autosomal manner and EBS Mendes da Costa, which is an X-linked recessive condition. The latter thus affects boys only, but boys and girls can be equally affected otherwise.

At present there is no ante-natal diagnosis available apart from sampling the baby's skin at around 18 weeks of pregnancy. Genetic counselling is advisable if there is a family history of the condition.

Characteristics

This condition affects only the **skin** and can clinically be divided into a 'simple' type, and a 'dystrophic' type depending on which layer of the skin is involved. Both types result in blistering from minimal injury.

In the **simple** type there is a wide variation in the degree of injury which produces blistering. Some babies may arrive in the world with a blistered skin due to the trauma of delivery. In others it is not until the crawling stage that any problems are encountered. In the latter circumstance, the movements of clothing on knees and elbows in particular when crawling is sufficient to cause blistering. Scarring does not occur in this type.

In the **dystrophic** type the degree of trauma again varies very much from individual to individual. Scarring is the usual outcome after healing in this type of EBS and can be severe, giving rise to contractures and maybe loss of finger- and toenails.

Depending on the sub-type, the blistering may occur anywhere on the body or be confined to the extremities.

The **mucous membrane** in the mouth may be involved in the young baby, but fortunately this does usually improve in later childhood. Soft, mashed foods should be given for as long as is necessary depending on the severity of the condition in the mouth.

Problems can arise when blisters become infected, and this can occur all too readily during the active 'into-everything' toddler years.

Other abnormalities can include the following.

Erosions and narrowing of the oesophagus which can give rise to difficulties with swallowing.

Contractures in the joints can also occur in some children with epidermolysis bullosa. This can cause a degree of disability later in life.

Management implications

The mainstay of coping with a child with EBS is the avoidance of **injury** as far as possible. The normal unavoidable bumps and falls of childhood cause greater problems than normal. Treatment of resultant blistering must be treated with great care to avoid infection. Children's skin differs from that of adults in that resistance to certain bacteria is less and so infection is a greater hazard. With increasing maturity, the blistering tends to improve and the susceptibility to infection diminishes.

School teachers should be alerted to the dangers to which their EBS pupils are exposed following even minor injury. Professional advice is a wise move if injury does occur at school. Teachers should remember that the usual sticking plaster for minor wounds should never be used on a child with EBS. On removal of the protective dressing, the abnormal skin will be painfully damaged.

An **adequate intake of food** must be maintained for the child with severe EBS. It is all too easy for nutritional deficiencies to arise due to eating problems in the early years. Children do not take readily to eating an adequate diet when their mouths are sore and eating is painful.

Some **sports** with much physical contact are unsuitable for children with EBS. Other activities, such as swimming, dancing and routine exercises are better for, and enjoyed by, these children.

Many everyday facets of life can be affected by EBS – for example, ironing can present a problem to the girl or boy with the disease, as the pressure needed to be exerted on the iron is sufficient in many cases to cause blistering with all its potential problems. Antibiotic creams will help reduce the possible dangers of infection in a blistered lesion to a minimum.

Tooth-cleaning can also cause blistering and soreness of the gums. A soft toothbrush should be used. Good dental care is vital, and teeth should be preserved in the mouth at all costs. The wearing of dentures in a sufferer from EBS is impossible.

Itching can sometimes be a feature of EBS, especially if the child becomes too hot. Avoidance of over-heating is important under these conditions, with perhaps an anti-histamine to reduce the irritation.

The future

EBS does tend to improve with maturity. Also sufferers, as they grow older, will learn how to avoid the injuries which they have found are likely to cause blistering.

Career prospects will be limited depending on the severity of the disease. For example, repetitive work needing the continual handling of objects will need to be avoided. Sheltered workshops, or suitable work from home, should be investigated for the EBS school-leaver.

Life expectancy is not diminished by EBS (except for the lethal form when death occurs in infancy.)

Self-help group

DEBRA
1 King's Road
Crowthorne
Berkshire RG11 7BG
(Tel. 0344 771961)

Aims and provisions: support and advice to sufferers and their families.

Fabry disease

Alternative names

Fabry–Anderson disease; angiokeratoma; alpha-galactosidase A deficiency.

Incidence

Due to the complicated inheritance pattern, the exact incidence of Fabry disease is unknown, but is thought to be about one in every 40 000 live births. All races have reported the condition amongst their populations, with the exception of the American Indians. The disease usually affects only boys; reports of symptoms in carrier girls are very rare.

Causation

Fabry disease is a metabolic condition in which there is a defective activity of a specific enzyme concerned with the metabolism of certain lipids in the body. As a result of this there is excessive deposition of these specific lipids in the walls of the blood vessels and also in other parts of the body. This in turn gives rise to the symptoms seen in this disease.

Inheritance of Fabry disease is as an X-linked recessive condition. There is a wide variety in the severity of the symptoms in each individual. Carrier girls can be affected but this is rare; again symptoms may range from completely absent to severe.

The condition can be diagnosed ante-natally by chorionic villus sampling, or amniocentesis.

Characteristics

The first signs of Fabry disease are usually seen in childhood. The child will complain of **pain** felt first in fingers and toes and then extending up the arms and legs, and maybe also across the abdomen and in the genital region. The pain is described as tingling or burning in character and can be very severe. The length of time for which these very unpleasant symptoms last also varies – from minutes to weeks. There may be a low-grade fever associated with each episode of pain. These painful events are often triggered off by excessive tiredness, an intercurrent infection or even by a rapid change in environmental temperature, such as coming into a hot room from a cold temperature outside. Children with these symptoms often will ask to go outside in the cold again. These periodic attacks of pain tend to become less frequent during adolescence and adult life. Many people with Fabry disease will complain of permanent discomfort in hands and feet. This often is said to be worse in the late afternoon and evening.

Skin: at around the same time as these unpleasant sensations occur, clusters of dark-red spots make their appearance – angiokeratomas. They can occur anywhere on the body, but most typically are seen in the greatest number in the lower part of the trunk and upper part of the legs.

Eyes: in later childhood, opaque areas, arising in whorls, are seen to be present in the cornea on examination under a slit-lamp. These will cause a degree of blurred vision depending on their severity. As well as these opacities, dilated and tortuous blood vessels can be seen coursing over the conjunctiva. On ophthalmoscopic examination, similarly damaged blood vessels can be seen in the retina.

Renal complications due to the involvement of the blood vessels of the kidney can occur in late childhood and early adult life. There is gradual deterioration of kidney function, and renal failure can occur at any time from the 10th birthday on.

Heart: the coronary blood vessels are also involved in the generalized abnormality due to the enzyme defect. This can result in coronary heart disease. Valvular heart disease – most frequently a prolapse of the mitral valve – is also associated more frequently with Fabry disease.

In a similar way, **strokes** can occur from damaged cerebral blood vessels.

Other more unusual symptoms can include:

1. nausea and vomiting, diarrhoea and abdominal pain due to depositions of abnormal lipids in the abdominal tissues;
2. Perthes disease due to avascular necrosis of the head of the femur;
3. delay in normal growth and in puberty in badly affected boys;
4. excessive fatigue and weakness throughout childhood in those severely affected;
5. chronic airway obstruction in severely affected children, due to the accumulation of specific substances in the lining of the airways, causing breathing difficulties.

The symptoms and signs of Fabry disease can be wide-ranging and severe leading to a good deal of difficulty in diagnosis. A firm diagnosis can be made by the finding in the blood of very high levels of the specific substances which are being incompletely metabolized.

Management implications

The **painful episodes** in limbs and other parts of the body can be relieved by giving certain specific drugs – carbamazepine for example. Other ways of helping children through these unpleasant symptoms is to be sure that they do not become too hot, and to try and avoid, as far as possible, sudden changes in temperature. Again, making sure that they do not get over-tired will help reduce the number of incidents of pain.

They can also be reassured that as they get older these episodes will become less frequent.

The **renal** and **heart** complications which can occur in later childhood need to be treated appropriately as they occur. Renal dialysis and kidney transplantation may be necessary in later life.

The future

Until kidney transplantation became available, death usually occurred in the forties due to renal failure. So life expectancy can now be prolonged unless the heart is severely affected, or a stroke is suffered.

Within the limits of disability, most careers can be followed, except those in which extreme ranges of temperature are found.

Enzyme replacement therapy is being researched, and in the future will perhaps, lead to a 'cure' for Fabry disease.

Self-help group

There is no specific self-help group, but the following group will give advice and help:
Research Trust for Metabolic Disease in Children (RTMDC)
53 Beam Street
Nantwich
Cheshire CW5 2NF
(Tel. 0270 629782)

Foetal alcohol syndrome

Incidence

Amazingly, this syndrome is said to affect to some degree one in every 100 babies born in Western countries. This incidence can vary from place to place depending on the drinking habits of the local population. If the drinking habits of the mother during pregnancy are very heavy, as many as one in three babies will be affected to some extent.

History

The specific characteristics shown by babies born to mothers who drink heavily during pregnancy have only been fairly recently described in detail. The amount of alcohol needed to be consumed before demonstrable effects are seen in the baby are not clearly determined. The result will also depend on both mother's and baby's susceptibility to the effects of alcohol.

Causation

Alcohol, and its derivatives, can cross the placenta, and so exert damaging effects on the developing child. The unborn baby not having available the enzymes necessary to 'detoxify' these substances readily will be susceptible to the adverse effects long after the alcohol has been eliminated from the mother's system. In addition to this direct effect, there can be other indirect problems. Malnutrition, dehydration and a poorly functioning placenta – all due to excess alcohol intake – can all add to the adverse effects.

   The developmental problems arise early in pregnancy, when maximum laying down of vital organs occurs – even before the mother herself is aware that she is pregnant. The severity of the problem will depend on both the timing during the pregnancy and the amount of alcohol taken. So it is important that drinking habits are controlled in all women who may expect to become pregnant in the foreseeable future. Defects due to this cause are probably one of the most obviously preventable of mental retardation.

Characteristics

Small size: babies who are born to heavily drinking mothers are often 'light for dates', i.e. they weigh less than would be expected for the length of pregnancy. Also they are frequently born prematurely. These babies are also slow to grow during the early months, not 'catching up' on weight and length as do most babies who are born before time.

Facial features are quite specific for babies born with the foetal alcohol syndrome. The forehead is narrow, with often small eyes and drooping eyelids which give a sleepy appearance. The top lip is long and smooth, without the 'rosebud' appearance common in babies. The lower jaw can be small.

Mental retardation frequently, but not invariably, occurs.

Many babies are **irritable** during the early weeks. Later they can become **hyperactive** and easily distractible. **Speech delay** has also been reported.

There is a wide range of these effects, but all children exposed to excess levels of alcohol pre-natally will show developmental delay and will probably not reach their full genetic potential.

Hearing may be affected, as there is sometimes specific malfunction of the Eustachian tube, that tiny tube linking the back of the throat with the middle ear.

Other possible effects are that babies have been noted to be very **hairy** at birth; **squints** are common; and increased susceptibility to **infections** of all kinds has been noted.

Management implications

Small size: children with the foetal alcohol syndrome will grow along the lower centiles of the growth charts, and there is little that can be done to accelerate growth. This persists throughout childhood.

Mental retardation: close watch must be kept on all aspects of development. Lagging behind in some aspects of the normal developmental process can be the first clue to diagnosis and so to subsequent development. Fuller assessment of areas of detected delay should be undertaken and appropriate help given to ensure that the child's full potential is reached. Speech therapy is frequently needed for speech delay.

Infections of all kinds, but most usually those connected with the respiratory tract, need to be swiftly and adequately treated whenever they occur.

Hearing must be routinely checked, and continued to be monitored on a regular basis, due to the potential Eustachian tube problems. This is especially necessary following a cold.

General care and nutrition of babies born to mothers with a drink problem must always be at the forefront of the health professional's minds throughout childhood. The mother may need help both to overcome her drinking problem and also to care adequately for her child. Health and social workers should cooperate fully to ensure that the child's safety, health and development are not adversely affected by a possible continuing drink problem.

The future

This is very much dependent upon the care received during infancy and childhood as well as the severity, or otherwise, of the alcohol effects.

Also, unless parents can be persuaded to give up their excessive drinking habits, the child, by imitation, can easily grow up into a similar pattern. Much education needs to be done on the adverse effects of heavy drinking during pregnancy.

Self-help groups

No specific group for mothers during pregnancy, but the following offers support and advice for people with drink problems:
Alcoholics Anonymous
PO Box 1
Stonebow House
Stonebow
York Y01 2NJ
(Tel. 0904 644026)

Al-Anon/Alateen Family Group
61 Dover Street
London SE1 4YT
(Tel. 071 403 0888)

Aims: Self-help for families and friends of those with a drink problem.

Fragile X syndrome

Alternative name

Martin–Bell X-linked mental retardation; fragile X chromosome.

Incidence

It is thought that mental retardation due to the fragile X syndrome occurs in approximately one in every 2000 to 3000 male births. This is very high figure, so this cause of mental retardation in boys is thought to be one of the most common. Girls are also affected, but to a lesser degree due to the mode of inheritance. Only 30% to 40% of girls carrying this genetic abnormality will have some degree of mental retardation.

History

In 1943 Martin and Bell first published accounts of a sex-linked form of mental retardation. In the late 1960s Lubs first described a family with the characteristics now known to be associated with the fragile X syndrome. The genetics of this abnormality have subsequently been demonstrated. Previously boys with mental retardation associated with few other physical features were termed as having 'pure' mental retardation.

There are a number of other syndromes of a similar type linked in some way to the X chromosome. Clinical features vary in these other syndromes, but mental retardation of some degree is a constant finding.

Causation

The cause of the fragile X syndrome is a defect in a particular part of the X chromosome (one of the sex chromosomes). This 'fragile' site is where the gene responsible for the disorder is situated. The actual genetic transmission is complicated and has not, as yet, been clearly resolved. Many families having a child with the fragile X syndrome show a definite X-linked pattern of inheritance, i.e. the condition being passed on from a carrier mother to an affected son. But many sporadic cases are now being recognized, or maybe they are variations of other X-linked syndromes.

At present there is no reliable ante-natal test, although chorionic villus sampling at 10 weeks of pregnancy can detect the fragile X syndrome in affected boys.

Characteristics

Mental retardation: the degree of this characteristic varies markedly from child to child. In some children the retardation is severe, whilst in others intelligence is on the borderline of normal. For example, there may be only mild difficulties with reading or mathematical concepts. But on the other hand, some boys can be so severely affected that characteristics such as hyperactivity, repetitive behaviour, autistic features, hand-flapping and speech difficulties occur. Girls with the fragile X syndrome – as confirmed by chromosome studies – usually have normal intelligence, although a few may be mildly retarded.

Testes in 90% of boys with the fragile X syndrome become larger than normal at puberty. This may affect one testis only. There does not appear to be any loss of normal function, although few affected men have been known to father children.

Facial features: a long, thin face is frequently associated with the fragile X syndrome in both boys and girls. Boys also tend to have large ears and a prominent forehead.

Other features can occur which aid diagnosis.

Speech is frequently specifically delayed during the early years. This can also be part of the general developmental delay seen as the child matures.

Fingers which are easily able to be hyperextended, due to the loose connective tissue around the joints, are also often a feature of children with the fragile X syndrome.

Skin is often fine and thin.

Management implications

All babies benefit from physical and verbal stimulation during the early growing years. This is particularly important for those children with potential **developmental delay**. Babies should be talked to from birth onwards, even though no obvious response is forthcoming. Similarly, simple games which encourage coordination of hands and limbs will help children develop to their full potential. Help in these areas is of particular importance to children with the fragile X syndrome.

Help from clinical psychologists can be of value in the early years if autistic or hyperactive behaviour is a problem.

Comprehensive multi-disciplinary assessment, on an ongoing basis, is vital to determine in which areas of development the child is lagging behind. Where problems are detected, appropriate help can then be given in the areas of delay.

Boys will probably need special schooling facilities, although this is not always the case, some boys managing mainstream schooling quite adequately, or, on occasions, with added help being available.

Again, full multi-disciplinary assessment is necessary to determine the most appropriate placement.

Genetic counselling for families who have a member with a proven fragile X syndrome is important.

The future

Career and job prospects will be limited in those boys showing the most severe mental retardation. Sheltered employment in a caring community or with full support from a loving home is the best option under these circumstances. For the less severely affected boys, and certainly for girls with this genetic abnormality, a wide variety of work is possible.

There is no limitation of life expectancy for children with the fragile X syndrome.

Self-help group

Fragile X Society
53 Winchelsea Lane
Hastings
East Sussex TN35 4LG
(Tel. 0424 813147)

Aims and provisions: support and linking of families; information and advice; promotion of research.

Friedrich's ataxia

Alternative names

Friedrich's disease; hereditary spinal ataxia; recessive spino-cerebellar degeneration.

Incidence

There are a number of conditions having ataxia as the prime characteristic. Friedrich's ataxia is thought to be the most common of the hereditary ataxias. Approximately every one in 50 000 babies born are likely to be affected. Boys and girls can be affected equally.

History

The most recent work on the basic cause of Friedrich's ataxia has been done by Harding. Suggestions have been made that the disease may be a metabolic one. This differs greatly from Friedrich's original thoughts on the matter, which were that the disease was due to alcoholic excess!

Active research into Friedrich's ataxia is currently being undertaken, and much work needs to be done to differentiate this form of ataxia from other conditions with somewhat similar symptoms.

Causation

Friedrich's ataxia is inherited as an autosomal recessive characteristic. The gene affected is situated on chromosome 9. The pathology is one of atrophy of specific parts of the spinal cord.

Ante-natal diagnosis can be made by chorionic villus sampling at eight to 12 weeks of pregnancy. Genetic counselling is advisable for families who have a member with Friedrich's ataxia.

Characteristics

Ataxia is the most obvious characteristic of this condition. At birth and up to around the age of three years there are no signs at all of any problem. In fact, the age at which the disease first manifests itself is very variable, and, in some children, symptoms only develop at puberty. The unsteadiness develops first in the legs, and ascends relentlessly up the body until all four limbs are affected. Accompanying this unsteadiness is weakness and an inability for the child to determine the position of his limbs in space. This fact adds to the ataxic problems. Sensations of touch are also diminished, but both pain and temperature change can be felt normally. Reflexes in the legs are lost early, and the plantar response is extensor. Regrettably, most Friedrich's ataxia sufferers will be wheelchair bound by the time they are 25 years of age.

Eyes: nystagmus or other disturbances of eye movements are noticeable in about half the children with Friedrich's ataxia. Optic atrophy also can occur in a minority.

Deafness, although less commonly seen than other abnormalities, can add to the problems of Friedrich's ataxia sufferers.

Scoliosis and **pes cavus** (flat feet) develop within a few years of the disease becoming obvious. These effects arise gradually over the years as the ataxic gait becomes more apparent.

Heart: the heart is always eventually affected in Friedrich's ataxia. This vital organ becomes hypertrophied (enlarged), and so functions less well. Breathlessness and palpitations are the symptoms most usually felt by the young person. ECG changes become obvious – left ventricular hypertrophy and T-wave inversion – as the condition progresses.

Diabetes develops in a significant proportion (20%) of people with Friedrich's ataxia, at a later stage of the disease. The development of this metabolic condition is more likely to occur in children, and young adults, in whom visual and hearing problems are in evidence.

Management implications

Ataxia: the child with problems of unsteadiness when walking will need to be protected against injury from falls during the early stage of the disease. Progressive weakness of the muscles will make many physical activities difficult or impossible. Depending on the severity, and rate of progression of the condition, a wheelchair will eventually become a necessity.

Physiotherapy, both to reduce as far as possible skeletal deformities and to keep weakened muscles on the move, is valuable. Many sufferers have commented that bed-rest seems to make their condition worse. So confinement to bed during any bout of intercurrent infection should be reduced to a minimum.

Speech therapy can be helpful in helping boys and girls to find the best way to use their muscles of articulation which are affected by the disease.

Vision and **hearing** must be monitored on a continuing basis. Any associated refractory defect or conductive deafness, due to infection, for example, should be treated early and adequately.

Heart: cardiac function needs to be accurately diagnosed clinically and by ECG, and maybe also by echo-cardiography. Digoxin and/or beta-blocker drugs are often helpful in maintaining adequate cardiac function.

Diabetes: the chances of this metabolic condition being strongly associated with Friedrich's ataxia must be remembered. Symptoms of thirst, frequent passage of urine and loss of weight must be urgently investigated, and appropriate treatment given if blood-sugar levels are found to be high.

Skeletal problems of scoliosis may be so severe as to need surgery. The deformed chest, due to the spinal 'twist', can give rise to problems with respiration.

The future

Friedrich's ataxia unfortunately pursues a relentless course with few, if any, periods of remission. Few sufferers remain out of a wheelchair by the time the early twenties are reached. A fatal outcome usually occurs before the fortieth birthday, most frequently from cardiac complications or an intercurrent respiratory infection. But these events can vary and life expectancy is enhanced for those people with less severe symptoms, and especially those with only mild cardiac symptoms and without diabetes. Improvements in treatment of cardiac and diabetic problems have, over recent years, also resulted in greater longevity.

Career choices are limited by the degree of ataxia, both affecting large muscle groups and the muscles of articulation.

Self-help group

Friedrich's Ataxia Group,
'Copse Edge',
Thursley Road
Elstead
Godalming
Surrey GU8 6DJ
(Tel. 0252 702864)

Aims and provisions: support and advice, together with fund-raising activities; leaflets.

Galactosaemia

Incidence

About one baby in every 50 000 born in the UK, the USA and Germany is affected by this metabolic disease. Ireland and Austria appear to have more babies born with this condition, whilst Japanese babies are affected very rarely. Both boys and girls can show the characteristics of galactosaemia.

Causation

Galactosaemia is inherited as an autosomal recessive condition. Chromosome 9 appears to be the chromosome on which the affected gene is located. Chorionic villus sampling at 9 to 12 weeks of pregnancy, followed if necessary by amniocentesis a month later, will show deficiency of the enzyme involved in this condition. It is the absence, or deficient production of, this enzyme that gives rise to the characteristic features. Galactose, a substance found in milk and milk products, is the substance which is incompletely broken down. So as a result, accumulations of this, and other allied substances, are found in various parts of the body in children suffering from this condition.

At birth the enzyme involved in the breakdown and proper metabolism of galactose is found to be absent when a sample of blood is taken from the baby. In the USA, all babies are routinely screened for galactosaemia by this method.

Characteristics

At birth the baby is entirely well. It is not until milk feeds are given on the second or third day of life that symptoms begin to appear.

The baby will, between four and ten days of age, become **jaundiced**, and begin to refuse his/her feeds. **Vomiting** will soon become a problem. As a result there will be a **loss of weight**, and the baby will become lethargic and drowsy.

One of the gravest dangers at this young age is that of **overwhelming infection** in any part of the body. Infections, particularly with *E. coli*, are particularly liable to afflict babies with galactosaemia. He/she will be gravely ill, and death is an ever-present threat under these conditions. Even if recovery does ensue from an infection, the baby's mental and physical development can be retarded unless the true cause of the problems are diagnosed and treated.

Cataracts can also develop in the eyes if treatment is delayed for too long.

Later problems can include specific **speech defects** and later **ovarian failure.**

Convulsions can also occur.

Treatment is by exclusion of all milk and milk products from the diet. If this is done early, within the first week or two of life, damage to the liver, brain and eyes can be avoided. If the diagnosis has been delayed, and milk feeds have been given for some weeks, jaundice, vomiting and loss of weight will become a grave problem. But once milk has been removed from the diet these symptoms will improve. Regrettably, however, the cataract formation, mental retardation and possible liver damage can be permanent.

Avoidance of all milk products must be maintained throughout life. There are a number of commercial replacements, such as soyabean products and casein hydrolysates, available which will satisfy the nutritional requirements of the baby. Normal physical growth can readily be maintained on these products.

Management implications

Early and adequate treatment of **infection** in the early days of life is of vital importance if the child is to survive. Special intensive care facilities may be needed for the babies that are very sick.

The **dietary aspect** of galactosaemia is the main problem to be faced once the baby has survived the first few traumatic weeks of life. Dietetic advice on suitable foods with which to replace galactose in the diet is a necessity for mothers and child carers. As the child matures it is somewhat easier from some points of view to avoid milk products. But the child may be under pressure from peers to try and eat, or drink, what they are eating or drinking. It must be explained carefully to the child, and to his immediate friends, that this course of action will cause him harm.

Speech defects do seem to be more commonly found in children with galactosaemia than in the general childhood population. The help of a speech therapist is necessary under these circumstances in order that understandable speech is learned.

Any possibility of **mental handicap** must be carefully assessed. Routine developmental tests should pick up any delay in any of the parameters tested. In this context, the speech delay common in this condition must be remembered. Early help with various skills in which the child has been found to be behind will be valuable. Teachers specializing in assisting pre-school children can be especially helpful. When school age comes around, assessment as to the type of school most suited to the child's abilities will need to be determined. Special schooling, or a unit with special resources may be necessary for some children with galactosaemia.

When reproductive age is reached, there may be problems of **fertility**. Female galactosaemia sufferers not infrequently have ovarian failure which renders them infertile. If pregnancy is achieved, genetic counselling and appropriate testing during the pregnancy are advisable.

Convulsions are not usual but, if present, will need to be treated with the appropriate anti-convulsant. Regular monitoring of any such drug regime must also be undertaken.

The future

Provided the exclusion of milk and milk products from the diet is begun early in the new-born period, and continued throughout life, there will be few problems – apart from, of course, the nuisance value of dietary restrictions.

Communication problems can persist into adult life in spite of appropriate therapy. So when career choices have to be made, it is wisest to avoid any career relying heavily on verbal communication. Infertility may also cause heart-ache.

Self-help groups

Galactosaemia Parent Support Group
31 Cotysmore Road
Sutton Coldfield
West Midlands B75 6BJ
(Tel. 021 378 5143)

Aims and provisions: contact with other families; information and advice about the condition.

The Research Trust into Metabolic Diseases in Children (RTMDC)
53 Beam Street
Nantwich
Cheshire CW5 2NF
(Tel. 0270 629782)

can also give advice and help.

Gilles de la Tourette syndrome

Alternative names

Tourette syndrome; multiple motor and vocal tics.

Incidence

It is thought that this distressing condition may be much under-diagnosed due to a variety of factors such as the varying severity of the disease, time of onset and social disability caused. Research has put the occurrence of the condition as high as between one in 2000 and one in 3000 for boys and between one in 5000 and one in 10 000 for girls. Boys would appear to be around three times as likely to be affected as girls.

Causation

Gilles de la Tourette syndrome is thought to be inherited as an autosomal dominant condition. But a high proportion of sufferers have no family history, so other factors may be involved. Birth injury, or the possibility of several genes being involved, are other suggestions as to aetiology.

There are no known means of diagnosing Gilles de la Tourette syndrome other than on clinical findings.

Characteristics

The age of onset of symptoms varies greatly, and can range from two to 21 years. The most frequent age at which problems become obvious is around seven years of age.

Tics: these are of two types.

1. Motor tics – involuntary movements of face, limbs and body. These unusual movements involve eye-blinking, facial grimacing, shrugging of shoulders and head and arm jerks. For a diagnosis of Gilles de la Tourette syndrome to be made these, and other, tics must be continuously present for over a year. Many children go through a stage where one or two tics occur, maybe copied from a friend or even an elderly neighbour! But these eventually are forgotten and are not replaced by other involuntary movements.
2. Vocal tics – coughing, sneezing, sucking, throat-clearing, sniffing and other unusual noises. At times the involuntary shouting of inappropriate words or phrases, including obscenities, can make life extremely difficult for parents and companions of the affected child.

These obscene words and phrases (including at times obscene gestures) occur in around one-third of all children and/or adults affected by this syndrome. This is a particularly socially disabling facet of the condition, and one which cannot be readily controlled. Vocal tics generally make their appearance some time after the motor tics have become established.

Obsessive behaviour is also a common feature of this syndrome. Repetitive actions and patterns of behaviour can be a further seriously disabling problem.

Reduced attention span can also make life difficult from a teaching point of view.

The whole pattern of Gilles de la Tourette syndrome is fluid and symptoms may vary in severity from week to week. Some particular problem may disappear for a time, only to reappear again at a later date.

Remissions can occur in some children, but usually the tics, both motor and vocal, and obsessive behaviour will reassert themselves again after a brief interval.

Management implications

Various drugs have been, and are still being, tried to reduce the motor and vocal tics. Results have been variable, but some success has been possible.

Schooling can be an especially difficult problem, due both to lack of concentration and to the difficult obsessive behaviour and repetitive multiple tics. Education may be necessary in a small unit where a variety of difficult behaviour patterns can be contained. It is of vital importance that the teaching staff are made aware of the diagnosis, so that appropriate care and teaching methods can be employed.

The future

Gilles de la Tourette syndrome is not a life-threatening disorder, but normal career prospects can be markedly limited by the symptoms. Social contact is also difficult, or even impossible, if the sufferer is severely affected.

Self-help group

Tourette Syndrome (UK) Association
2 Mark Close
Bexleyheath
Kent DA7 5JX
(Tel. 081 304 5446)

Aims and provisions: support and contact between individuals and families; promotion of research; newsletter and booklets.

Goldenhar syndrome

Alternative names

Goldenhar–Gorlin syndrome; ocular-auriculo-vertebral anomaly; first and second branchial arch syndrome.

Incidence

Studies on the incidence of this syndrome have only been recorded in the USA. In the Midwest of America one report observed an incidence of one in every 5600 live births. A further study reported an incidence of one in every 26 000 live births in the USA. There appears to be a slightly higher incidence of this syndrome in boys than in girls.

Causation

Patterns of inheritance seem to vary, and both an autosomal dominant and an autosomal recessive inheritance appears to be possible. The effects of the manifestations of this syndrome vary greatly, even within the same family. This makes both accurate diagnosis, and the sorting out of inheritance patterns difficult.

Ultrasound examination pre-natally may be able to detect ear abnormalities if they are present and severe. Other skeletal abnormalities, including the small lower jaw, may also be visualized.

Characteristics

Ears: Abnormalities in the anatomy of both the external and the middle ear are among the most obvious, and important, features. The size and shape of the external ear varies greatly ranging from virtually no external ear at all to a much misshapen pinna. This can occur in either one ear only or in both. The middle ear, containing those tiny bones vital for normal hearing, the ossicles, can also be tiny or misshapen. If these ossicles are small and/or misshapen, sound will not be conducted properly through into the nerves of hearing, and a conductive hearing loss will occur.

In conjunction with these abnormalities in the ear, the facial nerve can also occasionally run an unusual course. The Eustachian tube, linking the middle ear to the back of the throat, is also sometimes malformed. These defects can all add to the hearing problem.

Asymmetry of the face is a further feature in well over half of the babies born with this syndrome. The asymmetry becomes more evident as the baby matures, and by the age of around four years the unusual shape of the child's face is very obvious.

Cleft palate, with occasionally a coexistent cleft lip, can add to the unusual facial features at birth.

A **small, receding chin** can also be a characteristic. If this is present, difficulties with feeding can be worrying in the early days of life.

Eyes may be small with narrowing of the actual eyelids, making the eyes appear even smaller. About one-third of children with Goldenhar's syndrome have pinkish, yellowish growths, often containing much fatty tissue, associated with their eyes. These can grow to be as big as 10 mm in diameter. When they reach this size, vision can become obscured.

Other **skeletal abnormalities** can be present and wide-ranging, varying from unusually shaped vertebrae, which will eventually give rise to scoliosis, to abnormalities in the forearm and thumbs. (These latter features are reminiscent of the abnormalities seen in both the CHARGE and VATER associations. These two 'associations' of anomalies have somewhat similar defects in the forearm region. There is, however, no connection between these conditions and the Goldenhar syndrome.)

Heart defects occur with greater frequency than in other babies. Reports as to the incidence of this type of abnormality varies. Some authorities put the incidence as high as 58% of babies born with the Goldenhar syndrome. Ventricular septal defects are reported as being one of the most common of these heart abnormalities.

In a few children with this syndrome there may be some degree of **mental retardation**. Also, some children with very deformed faces can have severe **emotional problems**.

Management implications

In the early days of life, **feeding** can be a problem if the baby has a tiny lower jaw (cf. Pierre Robin syndrome). If there is also a cleft palate, with or without an associated cleft lip, this will add to the feeding difficulties. Tube feeding may be necessary in the early days to ensure adequate nutrition. The most severe cases can need surgical intervention for feeds to be given directly into the stomach. The unusual facial features can also lead to **breathing difficulties**, especially during sleep. A tiny lower jaw can allow the tongue to fall back into the throat, thereby obstructing breathing. Babies should be put to sleep on their sides to avoid this.

Hearing loss must also be diagnosed and fully assessed as early in life as possible to minimize the risk of delayed speech. The maximum age for the acquisition of speech and language is usually between one and two years. But before this time the baby is gathering information regarding various sound patterns by listening, especially to his/her mother. Any loss of hearing at either of these important stages can result in a much delayed speech ability. Once the hearing loss is diagnosed and treated as far as is possible, **speech therapy** input is valuable and often necessary for clear, understandable speech. As well as problems due to hearing, children with the Goldenhar syndrome can have difficulties in articulating their words due to their unusual facial features. Speech therapists have many methods of overcoming all these problems.

Eyes: if the typical growths are present in the eye region, they should be removed before their increasing size further precludes vision. Unfortunately, vision can also be adversely affected after this removal due to the scar tissue which inevitably forms following operation.

Cleft palate will need surgical repair if this defect is present. Surgery may also be needed for other facial asymmetries if they are severe and also amenable to this form of treatment.

Dental care is also important following the eruption of the teeth. Due to the asymmetry of the face, teeth will not always meet together properly, so orthodontic care will be necessary.

Heart defects, if present, will need assessment, and possible treatment depending on the type and effects which the defect is having on the child.

Mental abilities will need to be checked by routine developmental assessment at regular intervals, and assessment will need to be continued during the school years. Problems in any specific areas can thus be isolated and appropriate help given.

Emotional problems can arise particularly during the adolescent years if the facial disfigurement is very marked. Sensitive counselling and support from relatives and friends should reduce the impact of such problems to a minimum. Joining a group of similarly affected people can also do much to help.

The future

Life span is not restricted unless heart defects are severe or not amenable to treatment.

Careers may be limited in choice if there is any substantial hearing loss. Also facial disfigurement may be a factor precluding careers much in the public eye.

Genetic counselling when pregnancy is being considered as advisable.

Self-help groups

Goldenhar Syndrome Support Group
17 Andgowen Street
Greenock
Renfrewshire
Scotland PA16 8LG
(Tel. 0475 81263)

Aims and provisions: support and contact with other affected families; information leaflets.

'Let's Face it'
10 Wood End
Crowthorne
Berkshire RG11 6DQ
(Tel. 0344 774405)
is an organization which will also give support to people with facial disfigurements of all kinds.

Guillain Barre syndrome

Alternative names

Infective polyneuritis

Incidence

The true incidence of Guillain Barre syndrome is not known. There have been suggestions that the incidence in children has increased over the past two decades. The commonest time for the condition to occur seems to be in children between the ages of four and ten, although Guillain Barre syndrome is not unknown in babies. Both boys and girls appear to be equally affected.

Causation

There has been much discussion over the years regarding the cause of the Guillain Barre syndrome. As the condition frequently follows on from an acute infection it has been thought that it may be due to the toxic effects of this original infection. Hypersensitivity to some substance or organism, or the re-activation of a latent virus, have been other suggestions as to the cause.

There is no inheritance pattern involved in Guillain Barre syndrome.

Characteristics

Often Guillain Barre syndrome will start with **tingling** in the hands and feet. Along with these sensations will go severe pains in the legs together with tenderness when muscles are touched. This latter symptom is due to inflammation of the sensory nerves. All these symptoms can be of varying severity, ranging from acute pain to only intermittent tingling sensations.

Within a few days, legs will become markedly **weak**, and walking will be difficult. This weakness gradually extends up the body to the arms and, most serious of all, to the muscles involved with respiration. The young sufferer will feel generally unwell, and may have a mild fever, although this is often not a feature.

Symptoms will persist and may worsen for around a week or two, during which time the child is gravely ill. Admission to hospital is necessary and artificial ventilation may be needed to maintain breathing. Muscles around the face and throat can also become involved, making swallowing difficult, or impossible.

Once this acute stage is over, recovery begins. This is slow and can take many months before the young sufferer is fully fit again and able to use weakened muscles fully. Recovery is usually complete, and only a very small minority of children are left with any residual weakness. If this does occur, the disability is only minimal.

Management implications

Acute stage: once the diagnosis has been made, urgent admission to hospital is necessary. Intensive therapy facilities need to be readily available to ensure that respiration is maintained. There is no specific treatment available, reliance being placed on good nursing care, and maintenance of respiration should this become necessary.

Convalescence can be long, with paralysed muscles only slowly returning to full use. During this time, children will need adequate rest, a good diet and plenty of quiet pastimes available. Later on in convalescence school-work can be sent home so that too much schooling is not missed.

The future

Guillain Barre syndrome is a serious illness, but fortunately in the long-term the outlook is good with little or no permanent sequelae.

Self-help group

British Guillain Barre Support Group
'Foxley'
Holdingham
Sleaford
Lincolnshire NG34 8NR
(Tel. 0529 304615)

Aims and provisions: emotional support for people during recovery; public awareness about the disease; leaflets and other publications available.

Haemolytic–uraemic syndrome

Incidence

This is a rare syndrome, but one which can arise in clusters in different parts of the country. There are two quite separate ways in which this syndrome can arise, one of which is inherited and the other probably arising as the result of a viral infection. The exact occurrence is not known, but over 100 families having a member with the condition have been recorded. Either sex can be affected.

Causation

The hereditary form of this syndrome arises as either an autosomal dominant or an autosomal recessive condition. This inherited causative factor is thought to account for only about 5% of the known cases.

Other children, and adults, can suffer from the haemolytic–uraemic syndrome as a result of a previous acute gastro-intestinal illness. It can be difficult to distinguish the hereditary form of this syndrome from the acquired type. But there are two specific features which can point to one or other of the causative factors. Firstly, in the acquired form of the haemolytic–uraemic syndrome, symptoms of severe gastro-enteritis with bloody diarrhoea, and perhaps vomiting, are the early features of the condition. In the case of the inherited form, there is rarely any such preceding gastric upset – the characteristic features arising 'out of the blue'. Secondly, with the acquired type, other family members may go down with a similar illness within days or weeks of the first sufferer's illness. With the inherited form the interval between the onset of the illness in another related person can be anything between one and 14 years.

The haemolytic–uraemic syndrome can affect children (and adults) at any age from a few months onwards.

Whatever the causative factor, the features of the haemolytic–uraemic syndrome are similar, apart from the mode of onset.

Characteristics

Following on from the acute gastro-intestinal infection seen in cases of presumably infective origin, the following features occur.

Anaemia of a haemolytic type – the child will be pale, lethargic, feel unwell and tire readily on the slightest exertion. On checking the blood, the red blood cells are seen to be distorted and fragmented, and hence lose much of their contained haemoglobin (the oxygen-carrying substance in the red blood cells). The platelet count is also often extremely low. (Platelets are intimately concerned with the clotting of the blood.) Haemorrhages under the skin can arise as a result of these blood changes.

Renal failure can rapidly develop. Urine output may be much reduced, or there may be no urine passed at all. What urine is passed is seen to be blood-stained. The child is acutely and seriously ill, with perhaps very much raised blood pressure and cardiac failure. He/she will be restless and confused and convulsions can occur. Death can result during this very serious acute phase of the illness.

(The pathology behind these serious events is thought to be damage to the tiny blood vessels walls inside the kidneys. Following on from this, the blood cells are themselves damaged as a result of the rough, damaged blood vessel walls. A defect in the metabolism of a specific chemical, prostacyclin, has been suggested to be the prime cause of the haemolytic–uraemic syndrome.)

Following on from the acute illness, damage to the central nervous system (probably as a result of the convulsions which can occur), may happen resulting in a residual **mental handicap**. This is by no means always so, but must be remembered as a possibility. A recurrence of the acute illness can occur in some children at a later date. This particular occurrence is thought only to happen in those people who suffer from the haemolytic–uraemic syndrome which arises as a recessively inherited characteristic.

Treatment is dialysis to combat the acute renal failure. Blood transfusion will also be necessary to treat the haemolytic anaemia. This must be given with care so as not to overload the circulation, with the concomitant damaged renal output, with fluid.

Chronic renal failure may be the unfortunate end result if the acute stage of the disease is survived. This may require repeated haemodialysis, or continuous peritoneal dialysis. Kidney transplantation is the best long-term outlook.

Management implications

The **acute** stage of the haemolytic–uraemic syndrome will need intensive care facilities in hospital to combat the renal failure and possible hypertension and cardiac failure. Any succeeding recurrences of the condition will also be needed to be treated in a similar way.

Continuous ambulatory peritoneal dialysis may be the best way to treat a child with chronic renal failure following acute illness, whilst he/she is awaiting renal transplantation. Children accept this necessary treatment surprisingly well and become adept at coping with their unusual excretory process.

Mental handicap following from the acute illness must be recognized and subjected to detailed assessment. Some few children may require special educational facilities. If this is the case, ongoing assessment and help must be given.

The future

The outlook for sufferers from the haemolytic–uraemic syndrome is not good for those with the inherited form. Between 70% and 90%, in one report, were found to have died as a result of their illness, and 6% of the survivors were in chronic renal failure. Further attacks of acute illness may also occur.

Survivors of the acquired type may also suffer from chronic renal failure, or may make a complete recovery.

Career prospects will depend on the amount of residual handicap. Life expectancy will also depend on the severity of the after-effects. Genetic counselling is indicated particularly in those families in whom there is more than one member with the condition.

Self-help group

There is no specific self-help group associated with the haemolytic–uraemic syndrome, but the following organization can give reliable help and advice for renal problems:

British Kidney Patient Association
Bordon
Hants
(Tel: 0420 472021)

Haemophilia

Alternative names

Classic haemophilia; factor 8 deficiency; haemophilia A.

Incidence

The incidence of this well-known inherited condition is one in every 10 000 live male births (only boys are affected, due to the mode of inheritance). All races can be affected.

Haemophilia is a descriptive name used to describe a number of blood disorders which all have clotting problems as the basic defect. There are a number of 'factors' associated with the clotting mechanism of the blood. Haemophilia A is specific in as much as it is factor 8 which is deficient. Other factors are involved in the clotting disorders of other similar diseases, such as Christmas disease and Von Willebrand's disease.

History

Haemophilia has been known for many years, and is well-documented in history. Effective treatment was not available until the early 1960s. Previous to this, haemophilia was often fatal in childhood, or led to much disability and restricted life style.

Causation

Haemophilia A has an X-linked recessive inheritance. There is an abnormal factor 8 molecule in sufferers from this condition leading to the abnormal clotting mechanism. Between one-fifth and one-third of all cases are thought to arise sporadically as new mutations. The disease can be mild, moderate or severe. It is thought that there may be a different type of genetic inheritance in these three manifestations of the disease. About one-half of all known cases of classic haemophilia have the severe form of the disease. About 80% of sufferers have positive family history of haemophilia. The condition can be diagnosed pre-natally by fetoscopy.

Characteristics

All the features of haemophilia are entirely due to the defective clotting mechanism. The condition can be diagnosed at birth. Excessive bleeding from the umbilical cord can be the first clue as to the possibility of a bleeding disorder.

In severely affected boys, **haemorrhages** into joints are common. This occurs following only minimal trauma, or may be nothing more than the usual vigorous movements of joints common to all active children. Hips, knees and ankles in the lower limbs can all be affected as can wrists and elbows in particular in the upper limbs. This leads to **painful, swollen joints**, the excess blood inside the capsules of the joints causing the pain. Appropriate treatment must be given early to avoid damage and eventual destruction of the affected joints. Before the advent of specific treatment, grossly deformed joints due to degenerative arthritis was the inevitable result of frequent haemorrhagic incidents. This was especially evident in the weight-bearing joints such as hips and knees.

Bruising in soft tissues all over the body are commonly seen in haemophiliac boys. Again this results from only minor bumps.

In young children, bleeding from minor injuries to the **tongue** and **lips** is common. During the early days of learning to walk, falls are common and are often associated with damage to the mouth region. Inadvertent biting of the tongue is also common when learning to cope with solid food. Both these everyday events can lead to severe haemorrhage in the boy with haemophilia.

Bumps on the **head** are again very common during the growing years. This can result in disastrous bleeding into the brain in haemophiliac boys unless rapid treatment is given. This is one of the major causes of death in the young child with haemophilia.

In cases of suspected child abuse, the possibility of haemophilia – if not already known – must always be remembered.

(Less severely affected children will not be so vulnerable to minor injury. It is only when surgery, for example, tonsillectomy and other relatively minor procedures, are undertaken that the clotting defect is a problem. The more serious events, such as road accidents, that can be sustained by any child will also result in severe bleeding.)

Haemophiliac boys are especially susceptible to infection with **hepatitis B**. This can lead to progressive liver disease with a potentially fatal outcome. As soon as the diagnosis of haemophilia is made, immunization against hepatitis B should be given.

Treatment is by the giving of factor 8. Prompt infusion of this compound will limit the damage done by bleeding into joints. As soon as the bleeding occurs the treatment must be given. Some boys with haemophilia will develop a specific 'inhibitor', or immunity, to routine treatment. Subsequent haemorrhagic events will then need to be treated at a specialized haemophiliac centre. Some years ago, blood products used to treat haemophiliac patients were, regrettably, contaminated with HIV, and a number of sufferers have succumbed to AIDS as a result.

Heat-treated products, which render HIV non-infectious, are now used for treatment.

Management implications

It can be difficult to strike the correct balance in a boy with haemophilia between over-protection and lack of restraint. Parents will feel they must avoid even the slightest injury to their son with the resultant probability of severe haemorrhage. But, on the other hand, the child must be allowed to explore and investigate his environment as part of the growing process. It is all too easy for the boy with haemophilia to develop **emotional problems** as a result of his genetic inheritance. Support and advice from doctors, nurses and other professionals experienced in the handling of children with haemophilia is important.

Parents became very experienced during the early years in assessing the significance of any injury, and will also become adept at giving appropriate treatment.

Schooling will obviously present greater risks to the haemophiliac child. Teachers must be fully conversant with the action to be taken if a knock or other injury results in a bleed into a joint or other tissues. The telephone number of the haemophiliac centre responsible for the treatment of the child should be available in school. If in any doubt as to the action to be taken following an injury, advice can be obtained from this source.

Contact sports and other violent physical activities must not be part of the curriculum for the haemophiliac boy.

Education has an important part to play in the future career of a boy with this condition. Manual work cannot be contemplated, so intellectual pursuits and careers are of vital importance.

Care should also be taken in the use of aspirin in haemophiliac boys.

Von Willebrand's disease (or pseudo-haemophilia)

This is a condition which also has a relative deficiency in factor 8. Unlike haemophilia A, Von Willebrand's disease can affect both boys and girls, as the inheritance pattern is either an autosomal dominant or an autosomal recessive.

Symptoms of bleeding are much less than in haemophilia A. Nevertheless epistaxis (nosebleed) is common and bruising on minimal injury can result. In girls excessive menstrual flow can be a problem resulting in much discomfort and possibly anaemia. Excessive bleeding following surgery can also be a problem.

Treatment is by the giving of cryoprecipitate factor 8. Immunization against hepatitis B is also a wise precaution.

Later in life care must be taken in women to control bleeding following childbirth.

The future

With adequate quick treatment of bleeding episodes, the outlook is good nowadays for haemophiliac boys. Careers which include physical activities must be avoided, and body contact sports must not be indulged in as leisure pursuits.

Self-help group

The Haemophiliac Society
123 Westminster Bridge Road
London SE1 7HR
(Tel: 071 928 2020)

will be able to give advice and support.

Homocystinuria

Incidence

Homocystinuria is one of the rare metabolic diseases. As with other metabolic conditions, knowledge has vastly increased over the past decade into the biochemical nature of the problem. As a result of the screening programmes on new-born babies in most parts of the world, it has been found that Ireland appears to have one of the highest incidences of homocystinuria. In this country one in 60 000 babies are likely to be affected, whereas in Japan the number of babies with this particular metabolic problem has been estimated to be as low as one in 146 000. Both boys and girls can be affected.

Causation

Homocystinuria is inherited as an autosomal recessive condition.

Characteristics

Homocystinuria is a defect in the enzyme metabolism of specific amino-acids – homocystine and methionine. Excess homocystine is excreted in the urine and both homocystine and methionine can be found in excess in the plasma.

These two facts form the basis of the biochemical diagnosis and also result in the following features.

Skeletal system: children with homocytinuria are usually tall with long, slender fingers. (This, together with the similar eye problems, are very much the same features as are found in Marfan's syndrome.) Scoliosis may also be present, as well as knock-knees and chest deformities.

Eyes are commonly affected in homocystinuria, dislocation of the lens being the most common abnormality. Short-sight is also common and glaucoma and retinal detachment are further complications that can occur later in life. Appropriate treatment when, and if, these complications occur can reduce the incidence of severe visual problems.

Blood system: effects on the vascular system are the most worrying aspects of homocystinuria. Thromboses occur with greater frequency than normal, and can occur anywhere in the body – brain, heart, eyes, for example. Symptoms will occur in relationship to the part of the vascular system that is affected. (Due to this, venepuncture and surgical procedures should be avoided if at all possible, or certainly undertaken with great care.) This abnormal clotting can occur at any time of life, including infancy and childhood. The exact mechanism of this phenomenon is not fully understood.

Central nervous system: most homocystinuria sufferers have normal mental abilities, but a minority can show mild to moderate mental retardation. Early treatment does seem to help mitigate this. If thrombosis has occurred in the brain, this may also have a deleterious effect on mental abilities as well as the physical neurological signs. Convulsions can also occur, although this is comparatively rare, and, again, can be helped by appropriate treatment.

Management implications

Some cases of homocystinuria can be helped by treatment with vitamin B6 (pyridoxin), many features of the disease being improved; it is of vital importance that the susceptibility to treatment with pyridoxin is determined early so that various manifestations of the condition can be alleviated. The vitamin is given on a regular basis, and levels of the relevant amino-acids in the blood are measured regularly. If these levels approach normal limits, treatment is continued throughout life, with, of course, regular monitoring.

Folic acid supplements also appear to be necessary in some people with homocystinuria. This maximizes the good effects of the vitamin B6. A diet low in methionine can also be valuable, and the help of a dietician is of great value under these circumstances.

Eyes: visual acuity must be assessed regularly and corrective lenses prescribed for any refractive error found. The increased possibility of glaucoma and retinal detachment must also be borne in mind.

Vascular system: any thrombotic episodes, with the possible damaging sequelae, must be managed medically as they occur.

Central nervous system: children should receive regular developmental checks, with monitoring continuing when school-age is reached. Appropriate schooling can then be arranged should any problems be found. Checking of intellectual abilities after any central nervous system thrombotic episodes is also advisable.

The future

With appropriate early treatment in the vitamin B6-responsive type of homocytinuria, the outlook is good, and life expectancy is normal. Vitamin B6-unresponsive cases will have to rely on dietary measures as the sole form of available treatment. Under these circumstances, life-threatening thromboses are more likely to occur, but research is showing that early dietary restrictions, conscientiously adhered to throughout life, does improve the outlook.

Due to the increased risk of thrombosis it is not advisable for oral contraceptives to be used.

Self-help group

There is no specific self-help group, but the following offers help, support and advice to all sufferers, and their families, with metabolic disease:

Research Trust for Metabolic Disease in Children (RTMDC)
53 Beam Street
Nantwich
Cheshire CW5 2NF
(Tel: 0270 629782)

Hunter's syndrome

Alternative names

Mucopolysaccharidosis 2.

Incidence

Hunter's syndrome is an example of a defect in the metabolism of the complex sugars – the mucopolysaccharides. There are a number of syndromes in this group, and in each there is lack of a specific enzyme which controls the metabolism of these nutrients (Other syndromes include Hurler's syndrome, Morquio's syndrome and San Filippo syndrome.) Around one in 100 000 live births exhibit Hunter's syndrome. Due to the mode of inheritance of Hunter's syndrome, only boys have been known to be affected. All races of the world appear to have the possibility of being affected.

History

Until relatively recently, only seven mucopolysaccharide syndromes had been described – each due to a different enzyme defect. Recently however, 11 variants have been found, each with defective metabolism of a complex sugar. It is possible that further similar enzyme defects can occur.

Causation

Hunter's syndrome is inherited in an X-linked recessive way, so no girls are seen with Hunter's syndrome. Mothers carrying the characteristics can pass them onto their sons. The enzyme involved in Hunter's syndrome is a complicated one known as iduronate sulphatase. Due to the deficiency of this enzyme, mucopolysaccharides – complex sugars – accumulate in the organs and tissues of the body, where they give rise to the typical signs and symptoms of the syndrome.

Hunter's syndrome can be detected at around the ninth week of pregnancy by chorionic villus sampling techniques.

Characteristics

There are two types of Hunter's syndrome – one of which is milder and runs a less progressively downhill course than the more severe type.

These two types can be distinguished biochemically by the complex sugar which is excreted in the urine. It is the accumulation of this specific sugar in the organs and tissues which gives rise to the following characteristics.

Boys with Hunter's syndrome appear to have no problems at birth. They grow normally and pass all their developmental milestones at the proper time. During these early days the only noticeable problem can be noisy breathing which is frequently associated with a blocked and runny nose. But as this is often part of normal childhood anyway, no-one's attention is drawn to other possible problems. Head circumference measurements are within the upper limits of normal during these early years.

Umbilical, or inguinal, **hernias** are more frequently seen in babies who are subsequently found to have Hunter's syndrome, than is usual. But, once again, boys not having Hunter's syndrome can also have these weaknesses in the abdominal wall and so attention is not alerted.

From around two years of age onwards there is an obvious coarsening of the **facial features**. The boy's neck will be short, and his erupting teeth will be seen to be coming through widely spaced. Also over the succeeding months, these features are combined with a slowing down of the growth rate.

Joints can become stiff and the body is also often seen to be covered with a fine, downy hair.

At this time the **liver** and **spleen** becomes enlarged as a direct result of the accumulation of mucopolysaccarides in these organs. This enlargement can be a factor in the onset – or recurrence – of umbilical herniae.

Mentally, children with the mild form of Hunter's syndrome are of normal intelligence or only very mildly handicapped. Unfortunately, with the severe form, mental handicap is greater and will be obvious by around the age of eight to ten years.

As the boy matures, deposits of mucopolysaccharides can be found in many organs of the body – heart valves, coronary arteries, meninges and joints all being possibly included. It is one, or more, of these complications that will result in an illness with maybe a fatal outcome in a boy with Hunter's syndrome. For instance the damage to heart valves and/or coronary arteries gives rise to heart failure or, in the case of a blocked coronary artery, sudden death.

This clinical picture is very similar to that seen in the other mucopolysaccharidoses, although the basic genetic and biochemical faults are different.

Management implications

There is, regrettably, no curative treatment for Hunter's syndrome. Parents need sensitive counselling as to the future of their son, it being important to lay emphasis on the help that can be given to make life as normal as possible for their child – and themselves.

Herniae: if this weakness of the abdominal wall is present, this must be dealt with surgically. But (as in Hurler's syndrome), there is a high likelihood of recurrence due the further accumulations of muco-polysaccharides which increase the pressure inside the abdominal wall, so pushing the contents into weakened areas.

Hearing must be checked on a regular basis for children with Hunter's syndrome. Distraction tests suitable to the mental age of the boy will need to be done. Pure-tone audiometry is a further option, with evoked responses as a further aid to diagnosis where necessary. Deafness is common and hearing aids may be necessary later in childhood.

Contractures of joints, which can lead to grossly limited movement, can be kept to a minimum by physiotherapy. Hydrotherapy is particularly valuable and soothing. Therapy should be ongoing, with parents being involved in the treatment of their son as far as is possible. Sometimes surgery may be necessary to correct joint deformities.

Mental handicap in the severe type of Hunter's syndrome will need special education. Regular developmental checks are necessary to monitor all aspects of ongoing development in the boy with Hunter's syndrome. The results of such monitoring are necessary when decisions are being made as to the need, or otherwise, for special educational facilities.

With the milder type of Hunter's syndrome, normal schooling is usually satisfactory.

The future

Children with the severe type of Hunter's syndrome often only survive into their mid-teens to twenties. Cardiac problems, or severe respiratory infection, is the usual cause of death in the early or mid twenties.

Boys with the milder type of Hunter's syndrome enjoy a longer life span, and sufferers have been known to survive into their late sixties.

Children have been born to fathers with Hunter's syndrome. Families who have as a member a boy with Hunter's syndrome will need genetic counselling. Girls carrying the defective gene can be identified, and this is of crucial importance when pregnancy is being considered.

Self-help group

Society for Mucopolysaccharide Diseases
7 Chessfield Park
Little Chalfont
Amersham
Bucks HP6 6RU
(Tel. 0494 762789)

Aims and provisions: support and advice for parents; raise funds for research; annual parent conference held.

excessive thirst, frequent passage of urine or untoward loss of weight investigated urgently.

Problems of **obesity** are high on the risk factor list. Intercurrent respiratory infections can be dangerous for a very overweight Prader–Willi child.

A **fully independent life** is not usually possible for Prader–Willi sufferers, but work in a sheltered environment can be undertaken.

Self-help group

Prader–Willi Syndrome Association (UK)
37 Jasmine Close
Goldsworth Park
Woking
Surrey GU21 3RF
(Tel. 0483 676910)

Aims: to help parents and carers; to educate about Prader–Willi syndrome; to help research.

Primary ciliary dyskinaesia

Alternative names

Immotile cilia syndrome; Kartagener's syndrome.

Incidence

There are no exact figures for the number of people affected by this syndrome, but it is thought that as many as one child in every 4000 could be affected. Both boys and girls can suffer from primary ciliary dyskinaesia.

History

In 1933, Dr. Kartagener noticed the relationship between frequent chest and sinus infections and certain specific abnormalities of internal organs. This latter abnormality was the switching of position of some organs to the opposite side of the body. This could include the heart; this organ, under these circumstances, being situated on the right side of the chest.

In 1970, the basic problem causing the recurrent sinus and chest infections was found to be an abnormality in the cilia in certain parts of the body. (Cilia are the minute hairs to be found primarily in all parts of the respiratory tract, as well as in other parts of the body generally. Their function is to sweep secretions up and out of the respiratory tract. This is done by the cilia beating gently backwards and forwards.) In this syndrome the cilia are comparatively immobile. This effectively prevents mucus being removed from the respiratory tract. This static mucus then readily becomes infected, giving rise to the well-known symptoms of upper and lower respiratory tract infections.

Dr. Kartagener's original findings of the 'situs invertus' (internal organs on the incorrect side of the body) has been found to occur in only some sufferers from primary ciliary dyskinaesia.

Causation

This condition has recently been found to have an autosomal recessive inheritance. There is no diagnostic ante-natal test available as yet.

Characteristics

Commonly, babies with this syndrome will have some breathing problems at birth, due to difficulties in moving their normal secretions.

However, this quickly improves with appropriate neo-natal care. Often there are few indications that the child has any specific condition until the early toddler years, although the young baby is often noticed to have thick secretions constantly running from his/her nose. He/she may also suffer from a seemingly permanently blocked nose, which can cause problems with feeding.

During the toddler years, the child will be found to suffer from **frequent upper and lower respiratory tract infections**. Many children do, of course, suffer from frequent coughs and colds at this time of their lives. The child with primary ciliary dyskinaesia, however, will have an almost perpetually running nose, with thick mucus a constant problem. He/she will also have a constant loose cough. The upper respiratory tract infections will frequently extend down into the lungs, with the risk of resultant pneumonia.

Ear infections associated with these bouts of respiratory infection are also common. The thick mucus retained in the middle ear following these infections can also lead to a conductive deafness.

Sinusitis is again often associated with infections, causing headache and pain in the cheek regions.

Lack of a sense of **smell** is also a common associated problem. As well as missing out on a good deal of pleasure, the person lacking a normal sense of smell may not be alerted to the potential dangers of, for example, leaking gas and bad food.

Bronchiectasis can be the end result of the frequent lung infections. In this condition, the walls of the alveoli of the lungs are destroyed. This effectively reduces the oxygen-exchanging capability of the lungs, and also allows extra excess mucus to accumulate. These lung changes will only occur after a number of years of repeated infection.

Situs invertus is commonly present in children with this syndrome, but does not inevitably occur. The organs involved can vary; for example, only the heart (dextro-cardia – the heart on the right) being involved in some children. Other abdominally situated organs can also be reversed. Few symptoms need result from these anomolies, but occasionally added heart defects can also be present.

Symptoms of this condition vary, ranging from severe lung problems to only mild recurring chest infections, and the above anomalies may not be linked together for a number of years. But when it is realized that they may be connected, it is possible, by electron microscopy, to test the mobility of the cilia. A sample of cilia can be obtained by a nasal scraping. This test is expensive and requires skilled interpretation.

Infertility in men is one further problem associated with primary cilary dyskinaesia. The tail of the sperm has an almost identical structure to that of the cilia in other parts of the body. For normal fertilization to occur, this tail needs to be active. In primary ciliary dyskinaesia, this activity is much reduced. This results in the sperm being unable to move sufficiently for fertilization to take place.

Management implications

Antibiotic treatment, when necessary for severe respiratory tract infections, should be continued for an adequate length of time with maximal doses. Due to the thick secretions found in primary ciliary dyskinaesia, penetration by the antibiotics can be difficult.

Physiotherapy is valuable for the child who is severely affected and unable to cough up his/her sticky secretions. Postural drainage, two or three times a day, will help to prevent build-up of mucus and reduce infection to a minimum. This is especially important in young children, so that later bronchiectasis can be avoided. By the age of nine to ten years children can themselves learn techniques to clear their chests effectively.

Physical activities should be encouraged in children with this syndrome, provided that there is no other medical reason for avoidance of physical activity, such as a heart defect. Outdoor games and similar active pursuits are especially valuable.

Hearing should be checked regularly in all children who have associated frequent attacks of otitis media. If this occurs during the active time of speech development – between one and three years – there may be delay in acquisition of this skill. Following treatment of the hearing problem, speech therapy may be necessary under these conditions.

Myringotomy to drain excess fluid from the middle ear may also be necessary. Some authorities advocate the insertion of ventilation tubes ('grommets') to promote drainage of this fluid.

Heart defects, if present, will need appropriate treatment.

The future

This will depend on the severity of the ciliary abnormality. Some people will only be mildly irritated by their frequent nasal and sinus infections. Others will be frequently incapacitated by severe lung infections, and the effects of bronchiectasis. Due to these lung problems, smoking is inadvisable. The effects of the nicotine will inhibit he action of the cilia in the lungs even further.

Lack of a sense of smell, and a mild hearing loss, may pass unnoticed unless specifically asked about and/or tested.

Some men will be infertile due to this syndrome.

Life expectancy is not reduced, unless there are associated heart abnormalities, or the bronchiectasis is very severe.

Self-help group

Primary Ciliary Dyskinaesia (PCD) Family Support Group
42 Burstow Road
London SW20 8SX

Aims and provisions: lectures and information on syndrome; contact with families.

Retinitis pigmentosa

Alternative names

Rod-cone dystrophy; pigmentary retinal degeneration

Incidence

There is a group of conditions all classified under the name of retinitis pigmentosa. These all have a similar pathology in the retina – the light sensitive layer at the back of the eye. Modes of inheritance, severity and the age of onset of symptoms are the distinguishing factors between the different types.

Retinitis pigmentosa is also a feature of some other syndromes, for example, children with one of the mucopolysaccharide diseases (Hunter's syndrome) or with Usher's syndrome can also have retinitis pigmentosa as part of the problems encountered in their particular syndrome. Between one person in every 2000 and every 7000 is thought to be affected. Many of these people will have only minor visual problems; these can include poor night vision.

Both boys and girls can be affected, with the exception of the X-linked form of retinitis pigmentosa. Ante-natal diagnosis is not routinely available at present.

Causation

There appear to be three distinct modes of inheritance of retinitis pigmentosa. Autosomal recessive, autosomal dominant and an X-linked recessive form have all been described. As well as these inheritance patterns around half the cases of retinitis pigmentosa are the sole members of the family with the condition.

The autosomal recessive type appears to be the most common. This type first gives rise to symptoms during the first 20 years of life and progresses until the fifties or sixties when there is often severe visual loss.

The autosomal dominant type can appear early in the teenage years, but more frequently begins to give problems later in life, around 40 to 50 years of age. Progress is slower in this type.

The X-linked form is the least common, and, of course, only affects boys. This type is frequently the most severe and there will be severe visual disability by middle age.

These different types are thought to arise from different gene defects.

Characteristics

The basic abnormality in retinitis pigmentosa is a relative decrease in the number of 'rods' and 'cones' in the retina. These rods and cones are the light receptors which are a vital stage in the process of normal vision. In addition clumps of pigmented tissue can be seen in the retina. The tiny blood vessels of the retina also show degenerative changes.

All these changes add up, from a clinical point of view, to **reduced vision**. The amount by which vision is reduced is very variable, and some people will manage quite adequately, with only reduced night, and peripheral, vision. Often the first hint that a child may have retinitis pigmentosa is a complaint that he/she cannot see as well in the dark as his/her play fellows. A further sign is a narrowing of the amount that can be seen peripherally. (People with normal vision probably do not realize just how much they reply on their peripheral vision to make sense of the world around them. It is not until this is lost and virtual 'tunnel' vision becomes the result, that its importance is obvious.)

Colour vision is, at times, also affected.

Retinitis pigmentosa is not associated with other abnormalities elsewhere in the body. The exception to this, of course, is when retinitis pigmentosa is part of other syndromes such as Usher's syndrome or one of the mucopolysaccharide syndromes.

Management implications

Young children will not show any effects of their retinitis pigmentosa if they have the condition. But around 10 to 12 years of age their vision will deteriorate. Complaints of being unable to see the television or the blackboard at school clearly may be the first intimation that the child has a pigmented retina. Referral to an ophthalmologist will confirm the diagnosis when the retina is visualized with an ophthalmoscope.

Comprehensive vision testing is necessary to see if there is any degree of short-sight. This, and any other, refractive errors can be corrected by appropriate lenses, but no spectacles can help the basic problem in the retina.

Regular tests of vision throughout life are necessary to determine the rate of progress of the condition. In many cases this progression is slow and only in advanced years is blindness the result. A few children, however, may need special schooling facilities for their poor vision.

There are night vision aids available which can help with this aspect of retinitis pigmentosa.

In the USA, trials with vitamin supplements have been undertaken. There has been some suggestion that this treatment may slow the progression of the disease. But no conclusive proof has, as yet, been demonstrated.

The future

Careers which rely heavily on excellent vision, such as airline pilots, will not be possible for young people with retinitis pigmentosa. But, apart from those people who suffer from the severe, and rapidly progressive form, most careers will be possible. Life expectancy is normal for the retinitis pigmentosa sufferer. It is only when the condition is associated with some other, more serious, aspect (as found in other syndromes), that life expectancy is shortened.

Self-help groups

British Retinitis Pigmentosa Society
Greens Norton Court
Greens Norton
Towcester
Northamptonshire NN12 8BS
(Tel. 0327 53276)

Aims and provisions: information booklets available; fund raising for research.

The Royal National Institute for the Blind
224 Great Portland Street
London W1N 6AA
(Tel. 071 388 1266)

will also be able to give advice and help.

Rett's syndrome

Incidence

Rett's syndrome is thought to occur approximately one in every 10 000 to 12 000 female births. But recent research has shown that the condition is probably more common than was hitherto thought. It is now considered to be one of the commoner causes of retardation in girls. The condition seems at present to affect only girls, there having been no confirmed male cases.

There have been, so far, no biochemical or physiological abnormalities detected during life. Diagnosis is therefore entirely clinical. Definitive criteria have been agreed internationally.

History

The syndrome was first described by Dr. Andreas Rett from Vienna in 1966. There are a number of centres throughout the world who are now collaborating in research into this syndrome.

Causation

At present the mode of inheritance is uncertain, but, as girls only are affected, it would appear that there may be mutation of a gene on the X chromosome. The present hypothesis is that this abnormality is incompatible with life in the male embryo.

From post-mortem studies, the brain appears to be surprisingly normal, with no degenerative or storage disease apparent. But there is suspicion that certain areas in the cortex and basal ganglia may be affected. Evidence suggests that Rett's syndrome is a primary genetic disorder which only comes to light as development proceeds. This hypothesis fits the clinical picture. It is thought that some defect in the metabolism of noradrenaline and dopamine may cause this syndrome.

Characteristics

Following a normal pregnancy and birth, the baby develops within the accepted range of normal until around nine to 12 months, when **development ceases**. At this stage, the baby may be floppy, placid and show jerky movements. Then a period of regression sets in, with loss of the skills already learned. This stage may last for weeks only, but can persist for many months.

Speech: single words are usually developed, although it is rare for two or more words to be put together. During the regressive stage, these skills disappear.

Physical motor skills of both large and fine movements will be progressively lost. Walking becomes stiff and clumsy. Children previously able to feed themselves will lose this skill. As well as this loss of voluntary movement, involuntary hand movements such as frequent clapping, wringing and squeezing are very characteristic of Rett's syndrome.

Later, there is a tendency for **muscle wasting** to occur. Deformities of the spine and lower limbs can develop, with increased muscle tone. Some girls become chair-bound, but many women and girls can walk independently. Scoliosis can be made worse as a result of hypotonia and a sedentary life style.

These facts point to some disturbance in the central organization of movement in the brain.

Breathing: in many girls the breathing pattern is disturbed with hyperventilation alternating with periods of breath-holding. During these periods of disturbed breathing the involuntary movements of the hands are seen to increase.

Epilepsy may also occur. Abnormalities are seen on the EEG tracing, and are particularly in evidence in young girls when breathing is normal. This unusual finding is characteristic of Rett's syndrome.

Mental handicap is profound, and stable from around five years of age. The child is left with no speech and little self-help skill. Some communication can occur. Eye contact is good, and girls will respond to conversation.

Periods of crying are common during the regression stage, but usually decrease with age.

Management implications

Epilepsy: various drugs may have to be tried to control seizures if these are troublesome. Several different drugs, or combination of drugs may need to be given before a suitable one is found. Changes in the drug therapy may also be needed over time.

Mental handicap: children with Rett's syndrome will need assessment and subsequent admittance to schools for severe learning difficulties. Reassessment must be carried out on a regular basis to ensure that new needs can be met. Positive therapy in the form of structured training in life skills must be undertaken to prevent further deterioration.

Relative immobility can sometimes lead to **contractures** in joints. Physiotherapy is useful in the prevention of this. Hydrotherapy is valuable, and children enjoy this form of treatment.

All methods of **communication** should be tried. After 10 years of age communication skills, in some children, can be seen to improve. Thus, it is important that all possible channels of communication are kept open. It must be remembered that although sight and hearing appear to be normal in the Rett's syndrome girl, reaction times are slow. So, patience, understanding and a quiet environment are necessary to enable maximum benefit from skills training.

Music therapy has been found to be successful in controlling some of the extraneous movements of the hands, such as wringing, clapping, etc. Dr. Rett has worked extensively with children in this area of therapy.

The future

Children with Rett's syndrome commonly survive into their early forties. Occasionally some deaths occur suddenly and unexpectedly in mid-childhood.

Unfortunately, an independent life is never possible for sufferers from Rett's syndrome. But with careful supervision and behavioural training, a reasonable life-style can be attained.

Families, too, will need constant advice and support if the child is to stay in her home environment. Rett's syndrome is particularly distressing, as early development is normal. Day-centres and respite care can do much to support families.

Self-help groups

UK Rett Syndrome Association
Hartspool
Golden Valley
Castlemorton
Malvern Worcs WR13 6AA
(Tel. 068 481 357)

Aims and provisions: to offer families and carers support and friendship; to influence professionals and to further progress in fields of education, treatment and understanding of Rett's syndrome; to assist in research projects.

National Rett Syndrome Association
15, Tanzie-Knowe Drive
Camberlang
Glasgow G72 8RG
(Tel. 041 641 7662)

Reye's syndrome

Alternative names

Reye's fatty liver syndrome; Reye's disease

Incidence

In the early 1970s there were reports of a specific condition in infants and young children which, if they survived the original serious illness, could result in permanent handicap. Subsequently, much more has been learnt about the natural history of the disease. The number of children suffering from handicap due to this cause is not accurately known. In recent years, the incidence is thought to be decreasing. Children of any age, from infancy to around 19 years can be affected. The younger age group have been seen to be more at risk.

All races and both sexes can be affected by Reye's syndrome.

History

Reye's syndrome was first described by an Australian pathologist, Dr. Douglas Reye.

Causation

Reye's syndrome follows on from an acute viral infection, such as an upper respiratory tract infection, chickenpox, flu or a diarrhoreal illness. Various viruses have been implicated in these forerunning infections.

The use of aspirin to control fever and pain in young children with an infection has been suggested to be an added causative factor in Reye's syndrome. About 60% of children with Reye's syndrome have taken aspirin before the onset of the acute illness. As a result of this, aspirin is no longer prescribed for the relief of pain and fever in children under 12 years of age.

Recent research has suggested that some children who develop Reye's syndrome have an underlying genetically determined metabolic defect. This predisposes them to the symptoms seen in Reye's syndrome following an acute infection.

Characteristics

The **acute illness** is one in which persistent vomiting and convulsions follow on from an everyday, often mild, infection. The child becomes irritable and may be aggressive. He/she is confused and lacking in energy. Eventually, drowsiness can lead on to delirium and coma with a potentially fatal outcome. Bleeding from the stomach can also follow on from the persistent vomiting. Abnormal fatty deposits are to be found in the liver in association with encephalopathy (changes in the brain as a result of the illness) at post-mortem. The diagnosis can be difficult, as Reye's syndrome can closely mimic, for example, encephalitis, meningitis or acute poisoning. The child with any of these serious infections will, of course, need hospital treatment. Liver function and blood-clotting tests are necessary to confirm the clinical diagnosis.

The chronic phase: if the child survives the acute illness, recovery can be complete with no remaining permanent disability. But, unfortunately, some children will be left with a varying degree of brain damage. This may be only slight, but regrettably severe mental handicap can occur. If the infection affects babies under one year of age, there is more likelihood of residual disability than if this syndrome affects children over this age.

Management implications

Acute phase: urgent emergency treatment is necessary to reduce the risk of permanent brain damage. Early intensive treatment has been shown to increase the chance of survival, and also to decrease the risk of permanent brain damage. Intensive care facilities in hospital are frequently necessary in this acute phase.

Chronic phase: the acute stage of Reye's syndrome is a serious illness. The young sufferer will need several weeks of convalescence before he/she is fully fit again. Adequate rest, with a nourishing diet and graded physical activity will be needed. Many children will recover completely from their acute infection and suffer no long-term after effects. But regrettably some children will be left with permanent residual damage. The degree will vary, but in some cases mental handicap will be severe. If there is any doubt at all regarding possible brain damage resulting from the original illness, multi-disciplinary assessment will be needed. From the results of such assessment, any specific disability is unearthed, and so help can be given where necessary. In the most severely affected children, special educational facilities will be needed. Careful developmental follow-up over the succeeding years will be necessary. Any problem with movement, speech or cognitive function will need specialized help from the appropriate therapists. It is difficult to be more specific, as the after-effects of this illness are so variable.

The future

This will depend very much on the severity of the disability left once the acute illness is over. Recovery can be complete, with no sequelae. Alternatively, varying degrees of handicap can remain, affecting the remainder of the child's life. If this is the case, sheltered accommodation and work after special schooling facilities will be necessary.

Self-help group

National Reye's Syndrome Foundation of the UK
15 Nicholas Gardens
Pyrford
Woking
Surrey GU2 8SD
(Tel. 09323 46843)

Aims and provisions: support for parents; inform public and medical profession; raise funds for research to find the cause, develop early detection and improve treatment methods.

Riley–Day syndrome

Alternative name

Dysautonomia.

Incidence

This is rare in general populations. The Riley–Day syndrome is largely confined to Ashkenazi Jewish families. The incidence in these families is relatively high, being found in approximately one in every 3700 births. About one person in every 100 carries the gene. Boys and girls can be affected equally.

The Riley–Day syndrome is one which primarily affects the autonomic nervous system which controls the involuntary actions of the body, and functions such as blood pressure and temperature. In addition some voluntary movements, such as speech, swallowing and other physical movements can be affected also.

Causation

Riley–Day syndrome is inherited as an autosomal recessive. The incidence is relatively high in the population at special risk due to the comparatively closed community, with intermarriage being common. There is no ante-natal diagnosis possible at present. Genetic counselling is advisable for families who already have a member with the condition.

Characteristics

It is only the clumping together of a number of fairly non-specific symptoms in a child with a family history of the disorder that can lead to suspicions of the Riley–Day syndrome being present. All children with the syndrome have the following features:

No **tears** are ever shed by a child with the Riley–Day syndrome. This absence of tears can lead to ulceration of the cornea. Although there is some minimal tear formation in the tear glands, this is so defective as to leave no tears available to overflow onto the cheeks during everyday upsets.

The **tongue** in the child with the Riley–Day syndrome is smooth due to the absence of the papillae which are normally seen.

Other common signs affect up to 95% of children with the Riley–Day syndrome.

Blotching of the skin, due to the primary disorder in the autonomic system which controls the contraction and dilatation of the blood vessels. This is particularly noticeable when the child is excited.

Temperature control, also regulated by the autonomic nervous system, is unstable, and can become dangerously high or low. Excessive sweating, in an endeavour to lower a high temperature, is frequently seen in these children.

Pain is not felt as acutely as normal. This might seem like an advantage, but pain has the function of giving warning of injury or disease so that action can be taken to avoid further damage. If this built-in warning system does not function adequately, injuries can continue and disease processes can become dangerously advanced before treatment is given. The ability to distinguish between heat and cold is also often diminished – again increasing the risk of injury.

Incoordination of limbs when performing everyday activities is also noticeable in the child with the Riley–Day syndrome. In addition an unsteady gait is often seen.

Speech can also be adversely affected by the relative incoordination of the muscles of tongue and throat.

Scoliosis, together with general poor growth can also be a problem.

Intelligence is usually normal in children with the Riley–Day syndrome, but emotional instability is common, with wild swings of mood from elation to misery.

Blood-pressure control can also be unreliable. Hypotension is especially likely to occur when the child gets up from a lying or sitting position. This can cause temporary loss of consciousness at times.

Other less common, but nevertheless important, features include **swallowing difficulties** in infancy. This can make feeding a problem in the early days of life. **Uncontrollable vomiting** can also add to the problems of adequate nutrition in this age group of Riley–Day sufferers. Inhalation pneumonia is an ever-present threat when these two problems are encountered in infancy.

Management implications

Eyes: extra special care must be taken to protect the eyes of children with the Riley–Day syndrome. Dust which would normally be washed away by tears can cause serious abrasions on the cornea, with possible subsequent ulceration. So any foreign body in the eye must be treated with extreme care. Treatment with adequate washing out of the foreign body together with greasy, antibiotic ointment is a necessary precaution.

Infections of any kind must also receive adequate and early treatment, due to the instability of temperature control. This lack of control predisposes the child to febrile convulsions, so cooling measures must be taken as well as treatment of the underlying cause of the fever.

Pain insensitivity must be mentioned to teachers when schooldays are reached so that watch can be kept for any potentially damaging incidents.

Speech therapy is valuable in helping incoordinated muscle function of lips, tongue and throat.

Behaviour modification techniques may be of value in controlling the **emotional instability** which can be so destructive a part of the behaviour pattern of these children. The help of a clinical psychologist can do much to improve life for the child and his/her family. During anaesthesia, care must be taken with drugs which exert an effect on the autonomic nervous system.

The future

Children with the Riley–Day syndrome often succumb in early childhood to the effects of the swallowing difficulties which are part of their pathology – inhalation pneumonia often being the result. This can also recur in early adult life, with similar fatal results. Career prospects will be limited due to infections, possible poor vision due to previous unrecognized corneal abrasions and also to the emotional lability so frequently seen in people with this syndrome.

Self-help group

Dysautonomia Society of Great Britain
2 Oakwood Avenue
Borehamwood
Hertfordshire WO6 1SR
(Tel. 081 953 5900)

Aims and provisions: help with nursing problems; fund raising for research.

Rubinstein–Taybi syndrome

Incidence

This is a rare disorder, the incidence of which was reported to be only three affected in 100 000. This report related to the province of Ontario in Canada. Nevertheless, it has been estimated that as many as one in every 500 people in institutions for the severely mentally handicapped are affected by the Rubinstein–Taybi syndrome. This makes this syndrome a not insignificant cause of severe mental retardation. Because of the variability of the characteristics seen in this syndrome, the diagnosis can, at times, be made only tentatively. This further adds to the difficulties in assessing the incidence of the Rubinstein–Taybi syndrome.

The condition has been reported from many countries of the world, including Japan and Africa as well as populations of Caucasian origin. Both sexes can be equally affected.

Causation

The inheritance pattern of the Rubinstein–Taybi syndrome is uncertain at present. It may have an environmental cause as well as a genetic predisposition, or there may be a genetic cause as yet undetermined. Several sets of twins with the condition have been reported, and other familial connections are known. So these facts would make some genetic inheritance more likely.

There is no ante-natal test available to detect the condition.

Characteristics

Developmental delay is apparent in all children with the Rubinstein–Taybi syndrome. The delay affects all aspects of development, both mental and physical. The degree of delay varies from child to child, but the IQ will not be above 60 in the child with this condition. Along with the mental retardation comes varying degrees of language delay.

Microcephaly (head circumference at, or below, the lower range of normal). The head circumference measurement is an excellent indicator of brain growth, so it follows that all children with a head circumference smaller than usual will have some degree of mental retardation.

Physical growth in children with this syndrome is also retarded. Final height at 18 years of age will only be on the 50th centile of the standard growth charts.

There are a number of unusual **facial features** associated with the Rubinstein–Taybi syndrome, which make the children comparatively easy to recognize. **Eyes** are widely set apart, and eyelids have a characteristic drooping appearance (ptosis). **Eyelashes** are often beautifully long. **Squints** are also common, as are also **refractive errors**. The child's **nose** is an especially obvious feature, being on the large side and convex in a typical Romanesque manner. The mouth is small with, typically, a **high, arched palate**. **Teeth** are also often overcrowded, with an incomplete 'bite'.

Finger and **toe** features are among the most frequently found characteristics. Both thumbs, and nearly always also both great toes, are broad and flattened at the ends. The great toes are also widely separated from the other toes of the foot (cf. Down's syndrome). Occasionally, the terminal bones of thumbs and big toes are bifid, this feature adding to the broad, spatulate aspect of these digits. Other fingers can also be broader than usual at the ends. Toes can also overlap each other.

Other **skeletal** problems can also occur. For example, unusual construction of the lower vertebrae gives rise to an awkward gait.

In boys with this syndrome, undescended **testes** are frequently found.

Many children also have excess **hair** on their bodies.

There are a number of other abnormalities that can be associated with the Rubinstein–Taybi syndrome, including **heart defects**, **renal problems**, **convulsions** and **flame-shaped naevi** on foreheads or backs of necks. It is unusual for all these features to be found in one individual, but they occur with sufficient regularity to make remembrance of them necessary when caring for a child with this syndrome.

Management implications

Developmental delay, and all its educational and social effects, must be assessed and regularly monitored by a multi-disciplinary team. Particular areas of delay, for example, speech, should receive appropriate therapy. Early teaching of self-help skills will help to give a better quality of life to both the affected child and his/her family.

Appropriate **schooling**, geared to the child's assessed abilities, will be necessary when school age is reached. Depending on local facilities, either a special school or a unit with appropriately resourced facilities will nearly always be necessary for the child with the Rubinstein–Taybi syndrome.

Squints and **refractive errors** (be they short or long sight with or without astigmatism) must be assessed and treated appropriately. Squints may need surgery to prevent amblyopia. Refractive errors, more common in children with this syndrome than in the general childhood population, will need corrective lenses. Most children with these errors, however mentally handicapped, will willingly wear their spectacles. They appreciate the added dimension of clear vision.

Undescended **testes** will need operative procedures to bring these organs down into the correct position in the scrotum. Malignant change or damage due to trauma are both risks if this is not done.

Surgery may also be necessary on **toes** if the big toe is so large and displaced as to give rise to difficulties in finding suitable shoes.

Children with the Rubinstein–Taybi syndrome can suffer from **urinary tract infections** more frequently than their peers. This is particularly the case if there are associated renal abnormalities. These infections must be recognized and treated with the appropriate antibiotic when they occur.

Convulsions, if they occur, must also be treated with anti-convulsant drugs.

Obesity can be an added problem in the later childhood years. This should receive dietetic advice and monitoring.

Teeth, if overcrowding and/or malocclusion are present, should receive dental care.

The future

Most children with the Rubinstein–Taybi syndrome will never be able to lead a fully independent life due to their mental handicap. Full-time care will be necessary for practically all individuals. Life span is thought to be within the normal range as long as there are no potentially life threatening heart or renal abnormalities present.

A specific type of brain tumour is more common in people with this syndrome, and this can have fatal consequences.

Self-help groups.

There are no specific self-help groups for this syndrome.

San Filippo syndrome

Alternative name

Mucopolysaccharidosis 3

Incidence

San Filippo syndrome is one of the mucopolysaccharide diseases. The mucopolysaccharides are complex sugars. The defect in San Filippo syndrome is a lack, or deficiency of, a specific enzyme which breaks down one of these complex sugars. Due to this, there is an accumulation of the particular sugar in the organs and tissues. It is this build-up which causes the signs and symptoms of the disease. There are at least four sub-types of this syndrome, but all are similar clinically. The sub-types are known as San Filippo A, B, C and D. The difference in these four types is in the actual enzyme involved. San Filippo A is the most common.

Around one in 25 000 live births exhibit this enzyme deficiency. Boys and girls are equally affected.

History

With advanced biochemical techniques, the specific enzyme defects which occur in all the mucopolysaccharidoses have been found. All these diseases have a similar clinical picture, with greater emphasis on certain specific signs and symptoms in each syndrome, due to the specific sugar metabolism affected. (See Hunter's, Hurler's and Morquio's syndromes.)

Causation

San Filippo syndrome is inherited as an autosomal recessive genetic defect. Even though the enzyme for each sub-type is different the end result is that excess heparin sulphate is excreted and also stored in large amounts in the body due to the deficiency of the specific enzyme.

The condition can be identified pre-natally by chorionic villus sampling at around the tenth week of pregnancy.

Characteristics

Children with San Filippo syndrome are normal babies at birth, and initial developmental milestones are within the normal range. At around two to three years of age, or maybe even later – at early school age, this normal developmental progress slows.

Mental and motor development: sadly, after the initial normal growth and development in all areas, between the ages of two and five years, there is rapid decline both mentally and physically. Most of the skills of self-help and intellectual ability are quickly lost. The child becomes agitated and upset by the smallest changes in routine. Bizarre behaviour patterns are also noticed, similar to those seen in older severely demented people. Within a relatively short time he/she is confined to bed due to his/her inability to walk or to control his/her movements adequately.

Sleep disturbances can often be a distressing feature of the San Filippo syndrome. Parents can become quite exhausted by their baby's unusual sleep pattern which includes frequent waking during the night.

Growth is slowed at the same time as the mental and motor skills are lost. Although the gross short stature of Hunter's and Hurler's syndromes is not seen, children with San Filippo syndrome rarely grow beyond the 25th centile on the standard growth charts.

Facial features: there is a mild coarsening of the features in a similar way to that seen in the other mucopolysccharide diseases, although, again, this is not as marked as in the other diseases with a similar background. Tongue and lips become enlarged out of proportion with the rest of the face, and head size also increases.

Frequent **upper respiratory tract infections** are also a feature of babies with this syndrome. This can, of course, add to the sleeping problems as the baby is distressed by his/her blocked nose and all the other unpleasant symptoms of a head cold.

Deafness is thought to occur later in childhood, due most probably to the frequent upper respiratory tract infections. Hearing can be difficult to check accurately due to the severe mental retardation from which San Filippo children suffer.

Joints: as in the other mucopolysaccharide diseases there is some restriction in the movements of the joints. This, together with the loss of other motor skills, leads to lack of mobility.

All these signs and symptoms can be directly traced to the accumulation of the specific complex sugar which is continually being laid down in the tissue, and particularly in the central nervous system in San Filippo syndrome.

Management implications

Once the diagnosis has been made with certainty, parents should be sensitively counselled as to the future. It is incredibly hard to watch your seemingly normal baby deteriorate in all ways so rapidly and completely.

Parents will need to be helped through the normal bereavement processes – denial, anger, guilt and final acceptance, for the loss of a normal child is as truly a bereavement as if the child had died.

Mental retardation: the first sign of the occurrence of the regression from continuing normal development is often unusual and unpredictably inappropriate behaviour. The formerly biddable child will not be amenable to following the normal well established routine of the household and will exhibit temper tantrums for no obvious reason. Previously well-known and practised self-help skills, such as feeding and toileting, will be lost.

During this stage, patience and understanding are vital, and parents will need to be helped through each problem as it arises. Respite care for short or longer periods of time are essential in order that parents can have a break to recharge their own batteries as well as to give a little time to the rest of their family. Eventually, schooling for severely handicapped children will be necessary.

Hearing should be attempted to be assessed. This in itself can prove difficult, and even if it is thought that hearing aids would prove to be beneficial, it is unlikely that the child will tolerate them.

The future

The outlook for children with San Filippo syndrome is bleak. Death usually occurs before the twentieth birthday is reached, the sufferer being bed-ridden in a severely demented state.

There have been attempts to replace the missing enzyme, but so far this has proved to be unsuccessful.

Self-help group

Society for Mucopolysaccharide Diseases
7 Chessfield Park
Little Chalfont
Bucks HP6 6RU
(Tel. 0494 762789)

Aims and provisions: support and advice for parents; raises funds for research, including grants; annual parent weekend conference; supplies specialized hospital equipment; booklets and leaflets produced.

Silver–Russell syndrome

Alternative names

Silver syndrome; Dwarfism – Silver–Russell type.

Incidence

The exact incidence of this syndrome is not known, but cases have been reported from many parts of the world. All races and ethnic groups seem to be susceptible, and both boys and girls seem to be affected equally. (However, there has been an 'X-linked' Silver syndrome described, which has similar characteristics, but which, due to the mode of inheritance, affects boys only.)

Causation

The mode of inheritance is, at present, not clear. Either an autosomal recessive inheritance or a dominant inheritance with incomplete penetrance has been postulated. Suggestions have been made that placental insufficiency may be a factor in the aetiology of this syndrome. This lack of adequate functioning of the placenta may in itself be an inherited characteristic.

Characteristics

Short stature: babies with the Silver–Russell syndrome are born smaller than normal. Growth throughout childhood usually follows along the normal growth lines, but at, or below, the third centile on the growth charts. A few children have been reported to show a 'catch-up' growth spurt around puberty so that their final adult height more nearly approaches the norm, but this is unusual.

Asymmetry is seen, involving either one complete half of the child's body, or a particular part, for example, a limb or part of the skull. The degree of asymmetry varies markedly from child to child. Often this aspect of the condition is not noticed at birth or during the early months of life. It is only later, when growth proceeds at a rapid rate, that the unusual development is noticed.

Advanced sexual development, particularly in girls, is a common feature of the Silver–Russell syndrome. Breast development, menstruation and adult distribution of hair can all occur earlier than is usual. These effects go alongside elevated levels of gonadotrophins in the blood and urine.

The shape of the **head** is also a noticeable characteristic among children with the Silver–Russell syndrome. Foreheads are wide and taper down to a thin pointed chin, giving the appearance of a triangular shaped face. One further feature of interest is that the anterior fontanelle tends to be later than usual in closing.

The **hands** of children with the Silver–Russell syndrome are characteristic in as much as they frequently have an inturning little finger (cf. Down's syndrome). Toes, too, can show minor abnormalities, such as webbing, between the second and third toes in particular.

Café-au-lait spots, similar to those seen in neurofibromatosis, are often seen, on any part of the body. These can vary in size from those only the size of a small freckle to pigmented areas of over 30 cm in diameter.

Children with this syndrome have often been noticed to **sweat** excessively.

The last three characteristics (in head, fingers and skin) are all variable manifestations of the Silver–Russell syndrome. It is the combination of the short stature, asymmetry of parts of the body, the small size at birth, and the precocious sexual development that are the constant findings. The other added variable factors are, however, helpful in making a diagnosis.

Management implications

There are two aspects of the Silver–Russell syndrome which can call for special help in childhood. The **short stature** and possible **asymmetry** of the skeleton can cause difficulties during school days. The short stature is not usually so marked that the child will need special equipment, as do children with achondroplasia. The asymmetry of the body, if severe and affecting a major proportion of the body, may need to be corrected with, for example, special shoes, to aid normal movement. Physiotherapy is valuable in helping the youngster use the appropriate muscles correctly to balance his/her asymmetry.

The **precocious puberty** may be upsetting to both child and parents. Sensitive explanation, and practical help in school to deal with the everyday aspects of menstruation, will help the child come to terms with her unusual sexual development. It is not much fun being different from your peers in the upper junior school.

The future

The degree of affected movement will depend very much upon the position and severity of the skeletal asymmetry, and career choices may be limited by this aspect of the Silver–Russell syndrome. People with this syndrome can expect a normal life span.

Self-help groups

Silver–Russell Support Group
17 King Street Lane
Winnersh
Wokingham
Berkshire RG11 5AP
(Tel. 0734 773272)

Aims and provisions: support via telephone and meetings.

The Child Growth Foundation
2 Mayfield Avenue
London W4 1PW
(Tel. 081 994 7625)

is also able to give advice and information.

Sjorgen–Larsson syndrome

Incidence

Although this is a very rare syndrome, it has been reported as occurring in many countries of the world. Extensive research into this syndrome was done in the 1950s in Sweden. In a particular region of this country the incidence of the condition, named after the two Swedes who performed the research, was found to be around eight people in 100 000. Both boys and girls can be affected.

There are a number of other syndromes which cause a similar skin rash, But Sjorgen–Larsson syndrome can be diagnosed quite specifically by the associated features.

Causation

This syndrome is inherited as an autosomal recessive characteristic. The abnormal gene responsible has not, as yet, been located. Carriers of the condition can be detected by the deficiency of a substance necessary for complete oxidation of a further chemical necessary for correct metabolism.

There is no ante-natal test available.

Characteristics

Skin: the most obvious feature of the Sjorgen–Larsson syndrome is the specific skin abnormality. Soon after birth the baby's skin becomes reddened. Within a few weeks this redness becomes altered to a typical fish-scale like rash (icthyosis). The skin is dry and 'scaly' to the touch. Parts of the body most severely affected are the places which approximate most closely together, for example, armpits, elbow creases, around the neck and also the lower part of the abdomen. These typical skin lesions will persist throughout life.

A further characteristic of the Sjorgen–Larsson syndrome is **spasticity**. This is usually confined to the lower part of the body. As a result of this around three-quarters of the sufferers from this syndrome are confined to a wheelchair for most of their lives. Legs are stiff with increased tone in the muscles. An increase in muscle tone is also often seen around the mouth region. This can cause difficulties in feeding, particularly in the early days of life, and also problems with the subsequent development of speech.

Mental abilities: almost all sufferers from this syndrome have some degree of mental handicap. Some children are only mildly retarded, having an IQ level of between 70 and 90. (This level is defined as 'borderline retardation'). Other children are severely mentally handicapped.

These three features are those which must be demonstrated before a diagnosis of Sjorgen–Larsson syndrome is made. As mentioned before, a number of other syndromes have icthyosis as part of their pathology, but only Sjorgen–Larsson sufferers have the added characteristics of mental handicap and neurological signs.

Eyes: in around one half of the children with Sjorgen–Larsson syndrome there will be a degeneration of parts of the retina. This can occur as early as two years of age. If this does occur, vision will be affected to a greater or lesser degree depending on the severity and location of the retinal degeneration.

Management implications

Skin: the dry scales of certain areas of the skin seen in this syndrome can be very uncomfortable to live with, due to the associated dryness. Soap, which has a drying quality, should be avoided when bathing children with this condition. Lactic, or glycolic, acid can be used to remove the dry scales gently. This will need to be done on a regular, continuing basis. Other greasy emollient creams can also be tried in an effort to reduce the dryness. The help of a dermatologist is valuable. Clothing will need to be carefully chosen so that the dry, scaly skin does not catch on fluffy fabrics. Natural fibres, such as cotton, are probably the most suitable. Children, as they grow older, can become acutely embarrassed by their scaly skins so unlike the beautifully smooth skins of their contemporaries. Clothing with long sleeves and high necks will do much to reduce everyday embarrassment. Teachers will need to be informed of the child's skin condition when school days are reached, so that explanations can be given to other class members when playtime arrive in the summer.

Spasticity: little can be done to relieve this tragic neurological abnormality. In the early days of life, feeding may need extra care due to the tight mouth and throat muscles. Speech, for the same reason, may show articulation difficulties. Speech therapy input from an early age will ensure that speech develops as normally as possible. If the mental handicap is severe this will, of course, give rise to greater problems in this – and other – areas of development. Regrettably, children with Sjorgen–Larsson syndrome will eventually become wheelchair bound due to their neurological abnormalities. Good nursing care will be vital to prevent pressure sores.

Mental handicap: It is of vital importance that routine developmental checks are done for these babies and children on a regular basis. Just because Sjorgen–Larsson syndrome has been diagnosed, this does not necessarily mean that the child will be severely mentally retarded; IQ may be bordering on normal. So when school days are reached it is important that the correct school for the child's abilities is chosen if he/she is to reach his/her genetic potential.

Vision: careful check on visual acuity should be continuous throughout life. Ophthalmic examination will show if there is any retinal degeneration present. Little can be done to improve impairment to vision from this cause, but with routine checks other refractive problems of long- or short-sight or astigmatism can be corrected by appropriate lenses, so reducing the visual disability to a minimum.

The future

This is very dependent upon the severity of the neurological and mental disabilities. Life expectancy can be reduced if either of these two aspects is severe.

Self-help group

There is no specific self-help group in this country at present.

Soto's syndrome

Alternative name

Cerebral gigantism

Incidence

Soto's syndrome is a rare genetic growth disorder, the true incidence of which is not recorded, but 150 cases have been reported since 1964. Boys and girls are equally affected.

History

Dr. Jaeken in 1972 reviewed 80 children with the collection of characteristics which make up Soto's syndrome.

Causation

Soto's syndrome is thought to be genetically determined. An autosomal dominant pattern is probable, as evidenced by some families having more than one member with the same condition. Otherwise inheritance is sporadic due to new mutation.

The underlying cause is thought to be a non-progressive abnormality in the hypothalamic region of the brain.

Characteristics

Early rapid **growth** is the most obvious and consistent feature of Soto's syndrome. At birth Soto's syndrome babies are usually well up over the 90th centile for length. Growth is rapid throughout the first four or five years of life. Following this time, growth slows, but still persists along the upper ranges of normal. Final adult height is similarly in the upper ranges of normality, with only a very few exceptionally tall adults being recorded.

The **bone age** in children with Soto's syndrome is also advanced.

Tooth eruption and development is also advanced in line with the other bony characteristics.

Facial features: children with Soto's syndrome have a large head with a particularly prominent forehead. Eyes are downward slanting and are set wide apart. The chin is large and a high arched palate is also a feature.

Limbs: hands and feet in Soto's syndrome are also proportionately large. The arm span frequently can be greater than the child's height!

Mental retardation: although by no means invariable, between 50% and 80% (according to different authorities) of Soto's syndrome children have some degree of mental retardation. This is generally only mild, but some children are severely retarded.

Other more variable characteristics include the followings.

Seizures occasionally occur in this syndrome.

Renal tumours (especially Wilm's tumour) have been reported to have a higher incidence than normal in children with Soto's syndrome.

Clumsiness is evident in many children with this syndrome. This may be part of the underlying cause of the condition, but could be merely due to the rapid growth which occurs during the early years.

Management implications

Tall stature can cause problems in the pre-school years. Children with Soto's syndrome are both larger and stronger than their peers, and have not, as yet, learned how to control their strength and their actions. Hence, care must be taken that these children do not intimidate their playfellows. This can be especially difficult if there is also a degree of mental retardation. Strict supervision in playground activities, and guidance in suitable forms of self-expression will be needed.

Suitable clothing and footwear can sometimes be a problem in the three to four year-old child. He/she will require sizes more usually recommended for a ten year-old child.

Similarly, care must be taken not to expect too much, by way of ability or behaviour, from a child with Soto's syndrome. His/her size can belie the developmental stage attained.

Mental retardation: as part of routine developmental screening any persistently low scores in a variety of abilities in relation to age in a large child should alert carers to a possible associated learning problem. Full assessment of abilities in all areas of development will be necessary to determine suitable and appropriate schooling. Children with Soto's syndrome may need education for pupils with moderate learning difficulties, whilst others manage quite adequately in normal educational establishments.

Seizures, although not a common finding in this condition, will need to be investigated in order that appropriate anti-convulsants can be prescribed.

Wilm's tumour: the higher probability of this renal tumour occurring in a child with Soto's syndrome must be remembered. Most frequently the first sign is an abdominal swelling with no other symptoms.

Occasionally pain, or blood in the urine, are associated. Surgery, followed by chemotherapy and/or radiotherapy, is the necessary
treatment.

The future

Children with Soto's syndrome have a normal life span with few complications. As mentioned, Wilm's tumours must be remembered during
childhood.

   During both childhood and adult life, hypo- or hyper-thyroidism is a
possibility that must not be overlooked. Appropriate treatment for the
condition must then be given.

Self-help groups

Soto's Syndrome Society (an affiliate of the Child Growth Foundation)
2 Mayfield Avenue
London W4 1PW
(Tel. 081 994 7625; 081 995 0257)

Aims and provisions: advice and help to parents via telephone and
meetings; commissions research.

Sturge–Weber syndrome

Incidence

The number of people with this unusual syndrome is unknown, but it is thought to be a rare condition. Both sexes are affected equally.

Causation

The reasons behind the occurrence of the Sturge–Weber syndrome are also unknown. There does not seem, at present, to be any evidence that it is an inherited disorder. The most probable cause is a new mutation occurring sporadically.

There is no ante-natal diagnosis available, but the typical signs on the baby's face are obvious at birth.

Characteristics

A '**port-wine' stain** on one half of the baby's face is the very noticeable characteristic seen at birth. This specialized type of 'birthmark' follows the course of the fifth cranial nerve. This particular nerve is divided into three branches, supplying the forehead, cheek region and lower jaw respectively. The upper branch is most often affected in the Sturge–Weber syndrome, but all three branches can be affected so that the whole side of the face is covered by the purplish mark. The basic cause of this lies in an abnormality in the walls of the tiny blood vessels supplying the skin.

Parts of the blood supply to the **brain** may also be affected. On X-ray, specific 'tram-line' areas of calcification can be seen to appear when the child is over the age of two years.

Seizures are often a complication of this syndrome. The usual age of onset of these are after one to two years of age. This fits in with the altered X-ray appearance in the brain round about this age.

Sometimes **paralysis** of one half of the body occurs.

Both these latter characteristics are also due to the basic abnormality in the walls of the blood vessels which causes the naevus on the baby's face.

Eyes: At times **glaucoma** can occur in the eye on the same side as the port-wine stain. The narrow passage which allows the fluid inside the eye to drain becomes blocked by the blood vessel abnormality, and so cause tension inside the eyeball to increase dangerously. This condition, if not treated, can lead to blindness in the affected eye. Occasionally also the colour of the eyes may differ from each other. The eye on the affected side can be blue, even though the other eye is brown. This again is due to the abnormality affecting the blood vessels at the back of the eye.

Management implications

'Port-wine' stain: There is no easy treatment for this type of birthmark, particularly if it occupies an extensive area. Laser treatment is available in some centres, but this is time-consuming as only small areas can be done at any one time. Expense is also a problem. Cosmetic cover-up creams are available which give very good results at obscuring the mark, but these are more likely to be used later in life rather than in childhood.

Seizures will need to be treated with anti-convulsant drugs, and several may need to be tried before the right one, or combination of drugs, is found to be effective. If the fits cannot be controlled by medication, surgery to specific affected areas of the brain can be of value.

Glaucoma, symptoms of which are pain in the affected eye, blurred vision and possibly the seeing of green 'haloes' around sources of light, needs urgent treatment. Due to the blocking of the drainage ducts, tension in the eyeball is increased resulting in these typical symptoms. Treatment is by eyedrops or surgery. Without treatment, blindness can result.

Emotional problems can occur, especially in the teenage years, and also particularly in girls. Teasing about the facial disfigurement can lead children to become withdrawn. The help of a clinical psychologist will be helpful in the most severely affected children.

The future

This will very much depend on the extent, and sites, of the abnormalities in the walls of the blood vessels. If only the skin of the face is involved there is no threat to life or health. But if the disease is more extensive and affects other blood vessels in the brain, seizures can be a grave problem with potentially fatal results.

Self-help groups

Sturge–Weber Foundation (UK)
18 Wentworth Drive
Bromborough
Wirral
Merseyside L63 0JA
(Tel. 051 334 8171)

Aims and provisions: support, advice and information to affected families; promotes medical research.

Tay-Sachs disease

Alternative name

GM2 gangliosidosis

Incidence

This condition is usually only seen in Ashkenazi Jewish families, where the incidence is thought to be as high as around one in every 4000 live births. A further population group in which this serious condition occurs is French Canadians. Older children and adults are virtually never seen with Tay-Sachs disease, as death inevitably occurs in early childhood.

Boys and girls can be equally affected.

Causation

Tay-Sachs disease is inherited as an autosomal recessive. There are large numbers of people in the particular population groups mentioned above that carry the abnormal gene; the figure is thought to be as high as one in every 25 people. So, in spite of early death, there is still a great reservoir of people carrying this serious condition. Tay-Sachs disease is a further example of a condition which arises due to a specific enzyme defect. This deficiency allows certain chemical substances to build up in various parts of the body. These then given rise to the specific characteristics of the disease. The enzyme involved in this case is hexosaminidase A. The substance which is not adequately metabolized, due to lack of this enzyme, is a ganglioside.

Ante-natal diagnosis is available by chorionic villus sampling.

Characteristics

Tay-Sachs disease can be divided into two types, according to when the typical signs and symptoms make their appearance. In the 'infantile' type, the characteristic features begin to appear within the first six months of life. The 'late infantile' type (also known as Sandhoff's disease) will not show any sign of the typical features until the child is around two to three years of age. In this latter type two enzymes are involved – hexosaminidase A and B. In both types the features are the same, only the timing being different. All features are due to an abnormal storage in various parts of the body, but particularly in the grey matter of the brain, of the GM2 ganglioside.

Vision: In the infantile type of Tay-Sachs disease the baby of around six months of age will begin to disregard movements around him which had previously attracted his attention. An increased 'startle' response will be seen so that, for example, a person who has been nearby for some time will suddenly make him jump. Part of the reason for this increased 'startle' reaction may be, in addition to failing vision, a **hypersensitivity to sound**. This feature is one of the earliest signs that the disease may be present. On ophthalmic examination, there will be seen a cherry red spot on a particular part of the retina. This is a direct result of the build-up of ganglioside in this part of the eye. Within a very short time, the baby's vision will deteriorate so much that he will be quite blind, usually by one year of age.

Developmentally, loss of skills already learned is also an early sign of Tay-Sachs disease. The baby who will have been gurgling, smiling, lifting his/her head and moving arms and legs vigorously will become limp and unresponsive. This can be devastating to the parents who have been watching with delight their baby's increasing awareness of his/her surroundings. As with all the metabolic conditions, the deterioration of a seemingly normal baby can be almost unbelievable.

Seizures commonly begin to occur during the second year of life. Often, they will take the form of outbursts of quite inappropriate laughter. The EEG will show abnormalities in association with this event. These fits can be very difficult to control, and a number of anti-convulsant drugs may need to be tried before some degree of control is gained. As the disease progresses the episodes of seizures tends to lessen spontaneously.

Hypotonia, or a generalized weakness of all the muscles, rapidly follows on. The baby who previously had been rolling over and attempting to pull his/her head and shoulders into a sitting position will cease to try this. He/she will lie apathetically in his/her cot becoming more and more unresponsive to his/her surroundings. Only sudden loud noises will cause a 'startle' reaction along with the outbursts of laughter which denote a fit.

Eventually the baby's limbs will become stiff with exaggerated reflexes until a complete spastic paralysis results.

Head size can increase rapidly due to the deposition of abnormal material in the brain. This can give the appearance of hydrocephalus, although this is not the true cause of the increase in head circumference. (Hydrocephalus implies an increase in size of the ventricles in the brain containing cerebro-spinal fluid.)

The final outcome of this tragic decease is death by the age of three to four years. In the late infantile type (Sandhoff's disease) the characteristic features do not begin to make their appearance before two to three years of age. But a similar rapid deterioration as seen in the infantile type, proceeds, and death usually occurs between the ages of five and ten years.

Management implications

Support for, and explanation to, the parents is a vital part of this tragic genetic condition. Parents will need to have explanations given as to the inheritance of their baby's illness, the cause of the disease and the expected age of the final outcome.

Appropriate nursing care, together with help for parents on this aspect as long as it is possible for the child to be cared for at home, is virtually all that can be done. Eventually full time nursing care will be a necessity. Respite care, whilst the baby remains at home, so that parents, and any other members of the family, can have a holiday without the continuous worry of caring for a very handicapped child, is important.

Genetic counselling for couples considering a further pregnancy is advisable so that the risks of having a further child with the condition can be estimated.

Self-help groups

Tay-Sachs and Allied Diseases Association
17 Sydney Road
Barkingside
Ilford
Essex IG6 2DE
(Tel. 081 550 8989)

Aims and provisions: support for parents; promotes research; publications and information on screening.

The British Tay-Sachs Foundation
44a New Cavendish Street
London W1M 7LG
(Tel. 071 224 5185)

gives information on genetic counselling

Treacher Collins syndrome

Alternative names

Dysostosis mandibulo-facial; Franceschetti–Klein syndrome

Incidence

The number of people suffering from this particular syndrome is not known. A number of families with the disease, throughout several generations, have been described and researched.

History

In 1933, Dr Treacher Collins first described people with the particular characteristics seen in this syndrome, in a paper presented to the Ophthalmology Society of the UK.

Causation

This syndrome is inherited as an autosomal dominant. The penetrance rate appears to be high, but the degree to which sufferers are affected is variable. There is a high rate of mutations accounting for this syndrome – about half of all the cases described are thought to be due to this cause. Some of the babies born with Treacher Collins syndrome, having a new mutation as the cause, have fathers who are older than normal.

This syndrome has been successfully diagnosed pre-natally using fetoscopic methods. The specific characteristics have also been seen on ultra-sonic screening.

Characteristics

The abnormalities seen in the Treacher Collins syndrome solely affect the face and associated anatomical structures.

The bones of the **cheeks** (maxillae) are small and under-developed. This gives the false impression of a large nose, which is often initially the most noticeable feature.

The **lower jaw** can also be small, giving the appearance of a receding chin. This feature can lead to problems with respiration and feeding during the early days of life. During the relaxation of muscles during sleep, the tiny, under-developed jaw can drop back. This allows the baby's tongue to fall back into his/her throat and effectively obstruct breathing. This is especially dangerous if the baby is put to sleep on his/her back. The safest position for these babies is on their sides (laying babies to sleep on their tummies is thought to be a possible factor in the causation of the sudden infant death syndrome, and so should be avoided, even though it would appear to be an ideal position for the Treacher Collins baby).

Feeding, too, can be difficult due to the small jaw. A good 'seal' around nipple or teat is almost impossible to obtain until the baby matures and his/her lower jaw develops further.

Eyes have a downward slant at the outside edge, and this compounds the unusual features of the face. The lower **eyelids** may have a small gap, or 'nick' in their length (coloboma), and **eyelashes** may be absent on the nasal side of this feature. Fortunately this coloboma never seems to affect any other structures of the eye, as is the case in some other syndromes – the CHARGE association, for example. So there is no visual defect associated with the Treacher Collins syndrome.

Ears can be small and malformed. The internal parts of the ears, including the external auditory canal and the middle ear can also be abnormally developed. In around half the children with the Treacher Collins syndrome, a conductive deafness occurs as a result of these abnormalities.

Occasionally (in about 28% of cases) the baby with Treacher Collins syndrome may be born with a **cleft palate**. If present this will add to the early feeding difficulties.

A **heart defect** has also occasionally been found with this syndrome.

Due to the abnormalities possible in both upper and lower jaws, there may be problems with proper eruption of **teeth** at a later date.

Management implications

Early **breathing** and **feeding** difficulties, if specific abnormalities are severe, will need skilled specialized attention. Nasogastric feeding may be necessary if sucking is impossible in the first few weeks of life. A temporary tracheostomy may be necessary in the most severely affected children.

Surgery may be needed to repair a **cleft palate** if this is present. Also surgery may be necessary to repair some of the unusual facial features. Great improvement is possible with plastic surgery, particularly to the problems in the upper jaw.

The most important aspect of care for the child with the Treacher Collins syndrome is the early diagnosis of any **conductive deafness** that may arise due to the abnormalities in the auditory system. It has been regrettable in the past that children with severe hearing problems have been thought to be mentally retarded, with the result that both educational facilities and general handling have been inappropriate.

Hearing aids may be necessary from an early age, and this help with hearing will ensure that development is not delayed in other fields.

Orthodontic help may be required later on in childhood if teeth erupt crookedly.

Emotional support, especially if teasing at school occurs due to the child's unusual facial features, may be necessary for both child and parents from professionals concerned with the welfare of the family.

The future

Life expectancy is normal. A normal career choice is open to the child with Treacher Collins syndrome with the exception of deafness being a possible limiting factor for some careers.

Genetic counselling is advisable before pregnancy is embarked upon.

Self-help groups

Treacher Collins Support Group
114 Vincent Road
Thorpe Hamlet
Norwich
Norfolk NR1 4HH
(Tel. 0603 33736)

Aims and provisions: support and friendship for sufferers and their families; information by newsletter and reports on the syndrome.

A special group, dealing with all cases of facial disfigurement, is also helpful for families with a child with the Treacher Collins syndrome:

'Let's Face It'
10 Wood End
Crowthorne
Berkshire RG11 6DQ
(Tel. 0344 774405)

Tuberous sclerosis

Incidence

The estimated incidence of tuberous sclerosis is between one in every 30 000 to 40 000 live births. It is of importance as it is thought to account for 0.5% of all children with a significant mental handicap. Both boys and girls are affected equally.

History

Tuberous sclerosis was first recognized in 1880 by a Dr. Bournville, who described the pathological changes in the brain. Dr. Vogt in 1908 put together the triad of features, mental retardation, convulsions and the specific type of rash. In 1969, the genetic causation of the condition was described.

Much interest and work, particularly in the USA, has taken place over the past two decades. This has resulted in further understanding of the possible long-term effects of the condition.

The name, tuberous sclerosis, is derived form the tuber-like swellings which occur and harden (sclerosis) in various tissues and organs of the body.

Causation

Tuberous sclerosis can be dominantly inherited, but many cases are result of new mutations. Widely differing degrees of severity occur. In 1987, there was evidence that the gene for tuberous sclerosis is situated on chromosome 9.

There is no known ante-natal diagnosis at present. But if one or other of the parents is known to have the condition, ultra-sonic scanning can detect tumours in the baby's heart as early as the 20th week of pregnancy.

Characteristics

Infantile spasms may be the first sign to alert to a diagnosis of tuberous sclerosis. These are a very specific type of convulsions occurring in early infancy in which the baby bends at the hips a number of times in very rapid succession. (These attacks are also known as 'salaam' attacks). A characteristic pattern is seen on EEG. Affected children can suffer from fits throughout life.

Skin lesions of a specific nature may be the first sign if convulsions do not occur in infancy.

Appendix C
Glossary

Aetiology	The origin, causation and development of disease.
Amblyopia	Reduced vision due to squint.
Amniocentesis	Removal of amniotic fluid from around the foetus through the abdominal and uterine walls.
Amniotic fluid	Fluid surrounding unborn baby in the uterus.
Asymptomatic	No obvious signs of a disease process.
Ataxia	Loss of control of voluntary movement.
Atresia	Occlusion of a normal channel in the body,
Atrophy	Wasting of any part of the body.
Audiometry	Specialized tests for hearing.
Autism	Developmental disorder affecting communication and social skills.
Autosomal	Concerned with bodily cells.
Avascular necrosis	Death of tissue due to lack of blood supply.
Bronchiectasis	Lung disease following infection, often sustained in childhood.
Centile charts	Standardized growth (height, weight, head circumference) charts for children.
Choanal atresia	Congenital blocking of one, or both, nostrils.
Chorionic villus sampling	Pre-natal test performed on minute parts of placental tissue.
Co-arcatation	Narrowing of the aorta.
Colomba	Developmental gap in various parts of the eye.
Consanguinity	Close family relationship.
Dialysis	Method of removing waste-products from the body in the event of kidney failure.
Dyslexia	A specific reading difficulty.
ECG	Electrocardiogram, measuring the electrical activity of the heart.
EEG	Electroencephalogram, measuring the electrical activity of the brain.
Endocarditis	Infection of the inner lining of the heart.
Enzyme	Complex organic substance causing chemical reactions in the body.
Epicanthic folds	Folds of skin from upper eyelid over inner edge of the eye.
Eustachian tube	Tiny tube leading from the middle ear to the back of the throat.

Fistula	An abnormal connection between two organs of the body, or between an organ and the exterior.
Glaucoma	Raised pressure in the eyeball due to a fault in the drainage system.
Hernia	A weakening of muscular tissue allowing organs to protrude.
Hydrocephalus	Abnormal increase of cerebro-spinal fluid in the brain.
Hyperactivity	Extreme activity in childhood.
Hypertension	High blood-pressure.
Hypertonic	Increased muscular tone.
Hypertrophy	Excess growth of a particular tissue.
Hyperventilation	Over-breathing.
Hypoglycaemia	Low blood sugar.
Hypospadias	Abnormal opening of urethra on the penis.
Hypotonic	Decreased muscular tone.
Hypsarrhythmia	Particular type of convulsions.
Inguinal	Pertaining to the groin region.
Jaundice	Yellow colouration of the skin in liver disease.
Kyphosis	Bending of the spine in an anterior-posterior manner.
Lordosis	Normal curve of spine in region of the lower back.
Mainstream schools	Schools catering for majority of children.
Meconium ileus	Blockage of the small intestine in the new-born.
Meiosis	Type of cell division producing sex cells.
Metabolism	Chemical processes necessary to maintain life and health.
Microcephaly	A small under-developed brain.
Mitosis	Type of cell division producing similar cells.
Mutations	Changes producing new effects.
Myringotomy	Surgical procedure to withdraw excess fluid from the middle ear.
Naevi	Small pigmented areas in the skin – 'moles'.
Nystagmus	Jerky, sideways or vertical, involuntary movement of the eyes.
Parietal bones	One of the bones making up the skull situated at each side of the head.
Perthes disease	Disease of the hip in childhood.
Plantar response	Reflex action of the toes when the sole of the foot is stimulated.
Ptosis	Partial paralysis of the eyelids.
Reflexes	Involuntary responses occurring when specific parts of the body are stimulated.

Respite care	Short-term care, by paid volunteers, for handicapped children.
Scoliosis	Sideways bending of the spine.
'Situs invertus'	Organs on the opposite side of the body to normal.
Sporadic	Condition occurring in isolated cases.
Sprengal shoulder	One shoulder higher than the other.
Systemic	Condition relating to whole bodily system or group of organs.
Testosterone	Male sex hormone.
Thrombosis	Clotting of blood.
Tics	Involuntary movements of the face or body.
Tracheostomy	An artificial opening made in the trachea.
Ultrasound	Diagnostic test using ultra-high frequency sound waves to produce an image.
Urethra	Opening of the bladder to the exterior.

Index

This index should be used, in addition to the normal function, as part of the referencing structure of the book. For example, the distribution of 'deafness' or 'heart defects' amongst the various syndromes can be readily seen. The identification of a specific syndrome will also be more easily determined by referral to this index.

Puberty
    in Marfan's syndrome 146
    precocious, in Silver–Russell
        syndrome 195
Pyloric stenosis, and Noonan
        syndrome 160

Radius, in VATER association 222
Rectal prolapse, in Cystic fibrosis 66
Renal
    abnormality
        in Edward's syndrome 79
        in VATER association 222
    calculi, in William's syndrome 231
    complications, in Fabry disease 88
    failure, in Haemolytic–uraemic
        syndrome 113
    problems, in Lowe's syndrome
        142
    transplant, in Haemolytic–uraemic
        syndrome 112
Respite care 2
    in Aicardi's syndrome 15
    in Batten's disease 39
    families 6
    in Rett's syndrome 181
    in West's syndrome 229
Retina
    in Batten's disease 38
    in Usher's syndrome 219
Retinal detachment
    in Ehlers–Danlos syndrome 82
    in Homocystinuria 118
Rocker-bottom feet, in Edward's
        syndrome 79
Rod–cone dystrophy, *see* Retinitis
        pigmentosa

Salt, in Cystic fibrosis 65
Sandhoff disease, *see* Tay–Sach's
        disease
Santaveouri type, *see* Batten's
        disease
Scarring, in Epidermolysis bullosa
        84
Scheie syndrome, *see* Hurler's
        syndrome

Scoliosis
    in Aicardi's syndrome 14
    in Coffin–Lowry syndrome 56
    in Duchenne muscular dystrophy
        74
    in Ehlers–Danlos syndrome 82
    in Friedrich's ataxia 97
    in Goldenhar syndrome 106
    in Homocystinuria 118
    in Marfan's syndrome 145
    in Morquio's syndrome 152
    in Osteogenesis imperfecta 162
    in Riley–Day syndrome 186
Seizures
    in Angelman's syndrome 23
    in Coffin–Lowry syndrome 57
    in Prader–Willi syndrome 169
    in Rett's syndrome 180
    in Sturge–Weber syndrome 203
    in West's syndrome 228
    see also Convulsions
Sex organs, in Lawrence–Moon–Biedl
        syndrome 136
Shagreen patches, in Tuberous
        sclerosis 212
Sinusitis, in Primary ciliary
        dyskinaesia 173
'Situs invertus', Primary ciliary
        dyskinaesia 173
Skin
    in Cockayne syndrome 54
    in Ehlers–Danlos syndrome 82
    in Epidermolysis bullosa 84
    in Fabry disease 88
    in Fragile X syndrome 94
    in Riley–Day syndrome 186
    in Sjorgen–Larsson syndrome
        197
Sleep
    in Angelman's syndrome 23
    in West's syndrome 228
Small baby, in Foetal alcohol
        syndrome 90
Smell, in Primary ciliary dyskinaesia
        173
Spasticity, in Sjorgen–Larsson
        syndrome 197